the
CR
way

the CR way

USING THE SECRETS OF CALORIE RESTRICTION FOR A LONGER, HEALTHIER LIFE

PAUL McGLOTHIN & MEREDITH AVERILL
WITH ALISON HENDRIE

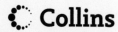

Collins

An Imprint of HarperCollinsPublishers

This book is intended to be informational and should not be considered a substitute for advice from a medical professional, whom the reader should consult before beginning any diet, exercise, or health regimen, and before taking any dietary supplements or other medications. The authors and the publisher expressly disclaim responsibility for any adverse effects arising from the use or application of the information contained in this book.

FIRST EDITION

Designed by Kris Tobiassen

Library of Congress Cataloging-in-Publication Data

McGlothin, Paul.
    The CR way : using the secrets of calorie restriction for a longer, healthier life / Paul McGlothin and Meredith Averill.—1st ed.
        p. cm.
    Includes bibliographical references and index.
    ISBN 978-0-06-137098-4
    1. Low-calorie diet.   2. Longevity.   3. Health.   4. Nutrition.   I. Averill, Meredith.   II. Title.

    RM222.2.M43467 2007
    613.2'5—dc22   2007030625

        09   10   11   12   WBC/RRD   10   9   8   7   6   5   4   3

CONTENTS

Part IV—Appendices

ACKNOWLEDGMENTS

We were in luck when we met Alison Hendrie, the extraordinarily talented writer who helped us create *The CR Way*. Her ability to quickly grasp CR science and transform our words into reader-friendly text was astounding. She also contributed text suggestions, organization, and was a great friend and manager for this project.

Working with Kathy Huck has been inspiring. Her amazing insights into what's important to the reader and how to organize the subject matter made a big difference.

Then there is Paul C. McGlothin, Paul's father, whose genius in biochemistry and pharmacology was the basis for Paul's training. His guidance, even to this day, helps us separate science fact from science fiction. Paul C's influence is felt on every page. Paul's mother, Joyce, lent her support and took time to read the text and give suggestions. Meredith's mother, Eva, who frequently gave us her support, saw the almost completed manuscript of *The CR Way* before leaving this world as the eldest member of the CR Society at ninety-five.

We were honored to have distinguished scientists review the text. How enriching to incorporate their comments into *The CR Way*.

Richard Lord, director of Science and Education of Metametrix Clinical Laboratory, used his powerful command of nutrition and biochemistry to review selected chapters and make suggestions.

Stephen Spindler, a world leader in CR research and our colleague in an upcoming genetic research project, was kind enough to review the CR science and make suggestions.

We are also tremendously thankful to be part of the great studies of human calorie restrictors by Luigi Fontana, John Holloszy, and their colleagues. The influence of these cutting-edge scientists is felt throughout *The CR Way*.

We also thank these talented associates whom we have the joy of working with regularly:

Jayne Jones, our dynamic office manager, who supported us with the things we needed to put *The CR Way* together page by page.

Pat Griffin, the brilliant cookbook connoisseur who used her experience and enthusiasm for cooking and cookbooks to analyze the recipes and improve their readability.

Matt Gross, our talented graphic artist who helped transform concepts into illustrations.

Elise Goyette and Harvey Light, who read sections of the book and came up with ideas to make it better.

Our doctors play such an important role in our CR life that we want to very sincerely acknowledge their contributions to *The CR Way*. Every one of them influences our approach to CR. In fact, the great internist, Dr. Abe Levy, himself a calorie restrictor, influenced Paul to start CR. We will be forever thankful for Dr. Levy's guidance.

Steve Bock, M.D., of the Rhinebeck Health Center and the Center for Progressive Medicine, raised our level of health, especially by analyzing our immune and elimination systems and helping us set standards for both.

Alphonse Aversa, M.D., the internist who oversees Paul's overall health, is like a good coach who readies his team: He helps Paul evaluate all systems before participating in calorie restriction research testing.

Jeffrey Powell, M.D., our endocrinologist, oversees our bone health, helps us develop hormonal evaluations of CR, and provides wonderful enthusiastic support for many of our CR endeavors.

Marc Grossman, O.D., a fellow CR practitioner and renowned optometrist, provides innovative guidance on eye health.

Monica Peacocke, M.D., a CR practitioner and former researcher, provides guidance to Meredith on gynecological issues and encouragement on CR matters.

Jane Geders, M.D., Ph.D., provides expert evaluation and advice on all gastroenterological matters, helps us develop standards to better evaluate colonic health, and provides help and support on CR.

Alan Schliftman, M.D., a superb dermatologist who provides whole-system guidance and innovative approaches that help us realize the tremendous cosmetic benefits of following *The CR Way*.

Stephen Abel, D.M.D., a wonderful artisan and dentist, has raised our standard for aggressive prevention of dental problems. He helps us guard against gingivitis problems that can ultimately derail the good cardiovascular outcomes produced by CR.

Working with this terrific team of supporters and influencers to create *The CR Way* has been a wonderful experience. It deepened our knowledge of CR and made the long walks we take every evening even more fun as we planned the text. We hope it improves your health and happiness as it has ours.

PAUL and MEREDITH

FOREWORD

Few things have captured the imagination of both the scientific community and the general population as the notion of extending life. Living longer, living healthier, living youthfully—these are widely desired goals. And today, they seem to be within our grasp.

Over the past several decades, calorie restriction (CR), a key to longevity, has stirred much excitement among researchers. It has been the focus of my research at the University of California, Riverside, for twenty years. Our lab has shown repeatedly that the rate of aging is strongly influenced by diet. The more calories an animal eats, the faster it ages. CR animals not only live longer, but they remain more active throughout life and remain free of cancer, diabetes, and heart disease for a much longer time.

After years of working with animals, CR science is now making strides in studying the effects of CR on humans. There are, of course, many differences between CR in humans and in animals, making the research link somewhat more challenging. In the lab, we subject animals to as few variables as possible. But people who want to benefit from CR do not live in such a controlled way. Our lives are complex. We are constantly subjected to influences that may affect our quality and length of life. Consider the many variables we sort through every day—positive and negative emotions, food selection, carcinogen exposure—all of which may affect how long we live.

As is the case with any scientific breakthrough, more research needs to be done and the CR concept continues to develop in stages. It seems as if we learn more literally every day.

Paul McGlothin and Meredith Averill have been at the forefront of CR for a long time. They were among the first to help organize and participate in the scientific exploration of CR in humans. In *The CR Way* McGlothin and Averill take the science of CR and craft a practical, easy-to-follow, and comprehensive action plan. *The CR Way* makes it possible for anyone—from the neophyte to the serious longevist—to follow their vision for a better and healthier life.

In addition to the potential health benefits of following *The CR Way*, my enthusiasm for this plan stems from the fact that everything the authors say is inspired either by their study of research results published in the CR science literature or by their own empirical testing. *The CR Way* lets you, the reader, take advantage of their experience—to practically apply the testing to your own life. This is invaluable information, and the authors are to be congratulated.

STEPHEN R. SPINDLER
University of California, Riverside

INTRODUCTION

Nobody expects to live forever. Staying healthy and strong well into our centennial years, however, is becoming an increasingly viable goal. The secret: When it comes to living a longer, healthier life, less is more.

Calorie Restriction (CR) is an approach to health and longevity that contends that consuming fewer calories daily than your body is accustomed to getting will increase energy, and improve physical and cognitive health, and may add years to your life.

It is science, not science fiction, that is demonstrating again and again the role of calories in the aging process. Excess not only leads to a larger waistline, it can also accelerate aging and promote illness and disease.

More than a dozen years ago, we read a remarkable article written by the eminent scientist Dr. Rick Weindruch on calorie-restricted mice that lived longer, healthier lives than other mice and on how to apply that research to humans. After reading the article, we were hooked. In the ensuing years, we've been developing—and living—*The CR Way*.

A vital point of *The CR Way* to longevity is to learn how to provide the body with less dietary energy, or calories, than it is used to getting. The body responds by learning to use the calories taken in more efficiently. The key to healthy calorie restriction is to eat nutrient-dense food—that is, food that has maximum nutrition per calorie, the opposite of empty calories.

You will naturally lose weight and body fat by consuming fewer calories on *The CR Way*, but this is not a traditional diet. Weight loss is a by-product of calorie restriction but not its main purpose. Our advice is to take it slowly. Remember, the emphasis of CR is to replace empty calories with fewer but more nutritious calories, allowing the body to maintain a healthy balance while removing the junk. Rapid weight loss can deplete the body of necessary vitamins, minerals, and other nutrients, as well as seriously compromise the immune system.

Some people believe that limiting calories would make you unhappy and dissatisfied, even if you did live longer. Others say it is simply too hard for most people.

That is exactly why we've developed *The CR Way*—a guide to longevity that incorporates a healthful lifestyle beyond just limiting calorie intake. This is not about sacrifice. It is about harnessing the body's own cellular signals to make every moment happier and better. You will eat food you love. You will discover reserves of energy you didn't realize you had. You will experience more good health and possibly more life to enjoy it.

Only a few years ago no one knew why calorie restriction slows aging and provides so many health benefits. Now, compelling new research shows that calorie restriction has important effects at the genetic level. These effects in turn affect the whole body's health. *The CR Way* is built on decades of scientific study and, more recently, research at the National Institute on Aging, Harvard University, Washington University at St. Louis, and medical laboratories around the world. Our own participation in numerous studies with many of these researchers has helped move the premise of longevity through calorie restriction from animals to humans, and from theory to reality.

Working with the distinguished lab of John Holloszy, at the

Washington University School of Medicine in St. Louis, our efforts have been to support research on the effects of long-term calorie restriction so that we can apply this knowledge to human health. The principal investigator of these studies is Dr. Luigi Fontana, a gifted medical scientist, trained in both internal medicine and metabolism. Already the research has yielded valuable insights that can be applied to humans.

Since calorie restriction is a relatively new practice, many of its methods can be misunderstood. We are here to help make CR more comprehensible and offer sound, practical recommendations about food, exercise, sleep—lifestyle choices that can improve your health and increase the likelihood that you will live longer. We also describe the beneficial effects of CR for people with diseases such as diabetes, cancer, and heart disease—as well as show how CR increases energy levels, concentration, memory, and an overall sense of optimism.

To assist in tracking your own progress along *The CR Way*, we've included easy-to-read boxes throughout, comparing the average test results of CR practitioners in the Washington University CR group to a group of people on a higher-calorie diet. These can serve as goals for you to improve your health. Be sure to always check in with your doctor, too.

The CR Way offers you a path to better health and the best chance for increased longevity. Let it be a road map to adapting your lifestyle by using this information in an entirely new way of looking at health and aging.

PART I

THE CR WAY

1

CALORIE RESTRICTION

The search for the fabled Fountain of Youth symbolizes the desire to remain young that has been a sought-after goal throughout history. It has been thought to be truly unattainable. Little did we know that the mythical waters of youth have resided within us all along. The human body is an amazing, resilient machine, shown to survive and thrive no matter what the external forces may be. Our evolutionary road has been a long, sometimes harsh one and yet we've adapted and flourished. How?

Researchers postulate that when our ancestors struggled through extended periods without food, the body's remarkable survival instinct would kick in and somehow slow down their aging. This allowed our species to live through difficult times—responding to hardships and challenges by becoming stronger and more resilient. The common thread appears to have been food, or rather, lack of food. The fact that consuming fewer calories somehow slowed the aging process has inspired scientific research for many decades. Most recently, science has begun to shine a light on what is happening on the genetic level.

Since the 1930s, when Dr. Clive McKay's breakthrough studies showed that calorie restriction greatly extended the lives of mice, scientists have been trying to discover how calorie restriction works. Thousands of studies have documented the broad range of health and longevity benefits of calorie restriction, but most theories on how it slows aging focus on only one of CR's many effects.

Calorie Restriction vs. Anorexia: The Facts

Although weight loss will naturally occur with CR, that is where any similaritity to anorexia nervosa begins and ends.

Anorexia is a clinically diagnosed psychological disorder characterized by distorted body image, excessive and unhealthy weight loss, and a fear of gaining weight. Individuals with anorexia often control their weight by all sorts of unhealthy actions, such as starvation, purging, extreme excercise, or other measures, such as diet pills. Anorexia is not practiced under a doctor's care.

Exactly the opposite, CR is both sanctioned and monitored by your physician with the purpose of living a longer, healthier life. By restricting calories while eating nutrient-dense foods, CR practitioners seek to activate the body's innate longevity system. As we caution in *The CR Way*, it should *never* be done to excess. Maintaining a Body Mass Index within the lower end of the NIH recommendations of 18.5–22 is fine for CR.

Rather than the self-destructiveness of anorexia, CR is all about building a positive, vital engine that will make your life better, happier, more productive, and, we believe, longer.

For example, identified effects of calorie restriction include:

- More effective disposal and renewal of cells
- Preservation of irreplaceable cells

- Reduced rate of growth
- More efficient energy production, including increased formation of mitochondria, the cells' energy generators
- Enhanced DNA stability
- Reduction of age-related decline of the immune system

Each is a positive health benefit and may contribute to longevity. However, a theory has emerged—hormesis—that explains these positive effects (and many others) of calorie restriction as the body's natural response to the low-level biological stress produced by reduced food intake.

HORMESIS

Just think about weight lifters who want to build their biceps. They determine a workout schedule with weights heavy enough to stress their arm muscles but not so heavy that they produce injury. The bodybuilders challenge the biceps with a form of hormesis, purposely pushing the muscle just beyond the standard, day-to-day activity to strengthen it. So we manage our amount of hormesis.

Now compare overeating to limiting calories intelligently: When you eat more calories or food energy than you need, your body often must cope with the added fuel by secreting insulin to process the high glucose levels circulating in your bloodstream. Some of the excess is stored for future use. But much of it is simply not needed, so it can end up being stored as fat tissue or deposited as plaque in your arteries. With so much food intake, your body does not need to use it efficiently, so your cells may run amok. Their job of reproducing themselves can be disrupted, sometimes resulting in unregulated cell reproduction that, in turn, can become cancerous cell growth. Your pancreas—the digestive organ that produces insulin—works overtime and becomes less able to do its job, and your heart beats more stressfully just to circulate blood to the extra tissue.

Stress That's Good for You

Some stress can kill. Researchers have shown that chronic psychological stress can significantly shorten the life span.

Beneficial biological stress—hormesis—has lengthened the life of laboratory animals by as much as 60%.

Calorie Restriction—A Beneficial Challenge

In contrast, when you limit your intake of calories intelligently, you challenge your body with a beneficial stress, or *hormesis*. With fewer calories available for energy production, your body shifts away from storing fat to actually using fat as well as protein for energy. Soon your cells produce energy more efficiently and your stamina increases. Meanwhile, cell reproduction slows—giving the body time to protect against mutations and preserving cells that may be irreplaceable. As

How Genes Work

Genes are regions of DNA that dictate the structure and function of organisms and control hereditary characteristics. Genes have their effect because they control the formation of proteins that have very specific regulatory functions within the cell. Many people think that heredity determines how our genes operate and that genes never change. This is only partly true. Some genes are activated or deactivated regularly by external stimuli such as dietary intake. This allows them to determine such aspects of our lives as how supple our skin is, how our muscles respond to exercise, and how fast we heal.

your body continues to adapt, you get stronger—becoming more resistant to disease and the deterioration caused by aging.

YOUR LONGEVITY SYSTEM

The incredible fact that humans have a survival system that can be switched on by the hormesis of calorie restriction came to light through a progression of discoveries at the lab of Dr. Leonard Guarente, at the Massachusetts Institute of Technology (MIT), in the late nineties. Research in 1999 produced the discovery of a gene—SIR2—that is activated by calorie restriction and promotes longevity. (SIR stands for Silencing Information Regulator, that is, a gene that regulates the deactivation or "silencing" of other *cell signaling*. Just as you send an e-mail message, your *cells* send information internally by electrical or chemical *signals*.)

Initially, many scientists considered the SIR2 "discovery" debatable. Later, work in labs around the globe corroborated that the SIR2 gene is conserved in many species, including human beings. So far, seven genes, a family called "sirtuins," have been discovered in humans and labeled SIRT1 through SIRT7 (Note: the *T* stands for 2 of SIR2, reducing the confusion of two numerals next to each other).

Of the seven sirtuin genes, SIRT1 is the most studied in mammals. It has been found that SIRT1 is activated by the stress of calorie restriction and that it silences a number of natural age-accelerating

Vitamin Caution

Your daily vitamin pill may contain a CR benefits stopper: According to several studies, nicotinamide, which is contained in many multivitamins, is an inhibitor of SIRT1.

triggers in humans, such as activation of growth-related hormones and increased inflammation. Sister genes SIRT3 and SIRT4 preserve cell life by facilitating energy production when calories are limited.

Our species might not have survived without the sirtuin family of genes to coordinate our hormesis response by shutting down the body's aging system when food is unavailable. We can use this capability directly by reducing the caloric intake into our bodies to trigger this survival mode, inhibiting our own aging systems.

GROWTH—A MIXED BLESSING

The miraculous process of growth helps you develop from a child to an adult. But it may also kill you. Just because you've reached physical maturity doesn't mean your body then shifts into idle. While SIRT1 may slow the rate of growth in some tissues, other growth regulators fuel the growing process throughout life and some may even accelerate it—contributing to the development of cancer and other age-related diseases.

The regulators our bodies need to grow don't necessarily distinguish between healthy growth and unhealthy—or cancerous—growth. In other words, the very hormones and cell signals that helped you grow from a child to an adult are the same ones that can fuel the growth of cancer. Lucky for us, these growth regulators are sensitive to what we feed them.

IT'S ALL ABOUT NUTRIENT AVAILABILITY

Many aging regulators have been discovered—some speeding and some slowing the aging process. What is important to know about these aging regulators is that they share a common "theme"—nutrient sensitivity. They are activated by more or less food availability, and some of those that accelerate aging are activated, independent of total calories, by high levels of glucose or protein.

BIOLOGICAL EFFECTS OF CALORIE RESTRICTION

CR consistently produces biological effects that are linked in laboratory animals to longer life. Understanding the "themes" of these biological effects helps enormously in practically applying the knowledge to lifestyle choices and in gaining maximum benefit from CR. Some major CR effects were identified in early research. More have been discovered in recent years. And we now know that we can affect many of them by our individual choices.

Here are the major CR effects that are important to understand when planning your journey on *The CR Way*:

- CR lowers circulating glucose and insulin levels
- CR reduces body fat
- CR lowers levels of growth stimulators
- CR prevents cell loss
- CR decreases inflammation
- CR creates a more youthful physiology

CR LOWERS CIRCULATING GLUCOSE AND INSULIN LEVELS

Blood glucose, also commonly known as "blood sugar," circulates through the body by way of the blood and lymphatic systems, and is the major source of energy in the body. When circulating glucose levels rise, the hormone insulin is released within minutes and helps glucose enter the cells. Insulin converts glucose into glycogen, the major carbohydrate reserve of animals. Additional insulin actions include stimulation of protein synthesis, formation of fat tissue, and increased cell growth. Sound like a 100 percent true-blue friend?

GLUCOSE AND INSULIN BOTH
ACCELERATE AGING

The more glucose you have circulating through your blood, the more insulin will be released to help regulate the blood sugar. High circulating levels of glucose and insulin are associated with accelerated aging and disease. In fact, high levels of both glucose and insulin have been independently documented as predictors of death rates.

Witness the staggering incidence of diabetes, a disease in which the body either fails to produce sufficient amounts of insulin, or is unable to use it properly to process the body's glucose. With more than 7 percent of the population of the United States, or 20.8 million children and adults living with diabetes, according to the American Diabetes Association, almost everyone is familiar with the frequent complications of Type II diabetes: Glucose levels that spiral out of control produce effects such as an increased incidence of cardiovascular disease, macular degeneration, nerve damage, and kidney disease.

JUMP-STARTING LONGEVITY GENES
WITH LOW GLUCOSE

Calorie restriction causes glucose and insulin levels to fall. The normal range for glucose levels—measured as fasting glucose, which is simply the level of glucose in your blood after you have not eaten for eight hours—is lower than 100 milligrams/deciliter (mg/dl). Calorie restriction will likely reduce this measurement. When glucose levels fall into the 80s or below, insulin production shuts down so glucose does not fall further.

Like a thermostat that turns on the furnace when the temperature falls, the SIRT1 longevity gene becomes active when glucose reaches this low level. This facilitates the burning of fats and proteins for fuel while reducing the risks of heart disease, inflammation, diabetes, and other age-related illnesses.

FASTING GLUCOSE LEVELS:
AGING-RATE INDICATOR

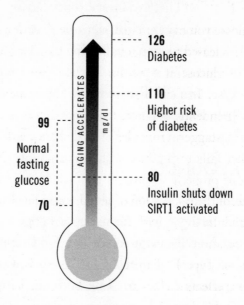

LIMIT CALORIES OR LIMIT GLUCOSE?

What is more important to *The CR Way*—limiting calories or limiting glucose?

Our answer: *Both.* While limiting calories lowers glucose and insulin levels—food choices, methods of preparation, meal timing and exercise can also profoundly lower glucose and insulin levels.

As with the biceps-curling weight lifter—the hormesis, or beneficial stress, we put on our bodies by restricting calories is enhanced by restricting our glucose levels. Low glucose levels may help jump-start the longevity gene, SIRT1, while keeping age accelerators like insulin at bay. We orchestrate our days to keep our glucose levels low—in the 80s or below for at least twelve hours a day. Using glucose levels as a gauge takes some of the guesswork out of how effective your longevity regimen is and provides a method of evaluating the hormesis you will experience. A simple, over-the-counter glucose test kit, or blood glucose meter—like those used by diabetics—will help you track your glucose levels.

If your glucose levels are high, don't be discouraged. When we first started calorie restriction, our fasting glucose levels were often averaging 90 to 105. But when we learned how important glucose levels are to activating SIRT1, we made achieving fasting glucose in the 80s or below a way of life.

ENERGY ABOUNDS

Some may think that CR's lower blood sugar levels mean that you would have less energy. Just the opposite happens: You will feel *more* energetic. As cells adapt to the low food supply, they create more energy producers, or mitochondria, and you will see the result: huge increases in stamina. Life becomes happier and more productive as your new high-energy state makes everything easier.

In a research study, healthy humans who followed a 25% calorie-restricted diet for just six months found that the diet helped make their bodies burn calories more efficiently.

- The overall calories they burned during a 24-hour period declined significantly.
- The number of their cells' energy producers, called mitochondria, increased.
- DNA damage, produced by oxidative stress from the production of energy, declined.

(Civitarese, 2007)

Cells will also use energy more efficiently, so the body benefits more from the smaller amount of food that's available.

How long you will travel *The CR Way* before you will see these changes depends on your body and all its history. We started to see beneficial changes within a few months. This mirrors findings reported in the scientific literature.

FRIENDLY STRESSORS

As we've shown with hormesis, "friendly" or beneficial stress does actually exist. The hormone cortisol, for example, increases blood pressure and blood sugar in response to stress. While that may sound bad, the fact is, calorie restrictors typically have high cortisol levels and benefit from them. In the morning, when fasting glucose is often at its lowest, cortisol raises circulating glucose levels while mobilizing fat stores for burning.

Another friendly stressor—epinephrine or adrenaline—which is known as the fight-or-flight hormone, is also higher in CR practitioners, where, like cortisol, it plays an important role in maintaining glucose levels. On *The CR Way*, you can learn through meditation how to channel the increased alertness that epinephrine provides into positive actions.

CR REDUCES BODY FAT

The CR Way is not meant to be a weight-loss or fat-reduction diet. But with the decreased caloric intake, the body naturally diverts existing body fat from storage to use as energy.

The average male has between 17 percent and 19 percent body fat, and the average female runs between 18 percent and 22 percent. Many CR practitioners have very low body fat, more comparable to Olympic athletes than to the general population:

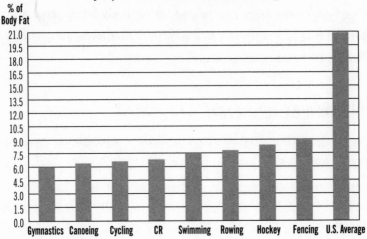

MALE BODY FAT
Calorie Restrictors Compared to Olympic Athletes and U.S. Average

Sources: J.E.L. Carter, 1982, L. Fontana, 2004, and University of Pennsylvania, 2005

High levels of body fat are dangerous. A survey of 850 men, aged 25 to 64, found a significant correlation between body fat levels and disease, particularly heart disease, hypertension, and diabetes.

Emphasizing how rare it is to find low body fat in the general population, the study found only 5 out of 121 in the 45- to 55-year-old category with body fat under 10 percent while all the Washington University study calorie restrictors of the same sex and approximately the same age had an average body fat of only 6.7 percent.

In calorie restriction, when SIRT1 is activated, one of the "villains" it shuts down is the fat-managing gene (PPAR gamma) that facilitates fat storage. By turning this gene off, fat accumulation and storage are also effectively turned off, allowing the body to burn fat for energy more efficiently. So what does fat have to do

A comparison of body fat percentages among Olympic athletes, calorie restrictors, and the average population eating a Western diet.

with longevity? A 2004 study by researchers at MIT has linked the reduction of fat deposits in mice to longer life. Scientists are still investigating what this means for humans, but in the meantime, there is ample research showing that lower body fat means a healthier you, reducing the risk for heart disease, diabetes, and other age-related diseases.

IS NO BODY FAT A GOOD IDEA?

Some suggest that fat reduction is central to calorie restriction's ability to lengthen life span.

But can it be a case of too *little* of a good thing?

A certain amount of fat is necessary because it regulates body temperature, protects and pads internal organs, and is the primary storage for the body's energy. But given the strong correlation between body fat and aging, some longevity enthusiasts let their body fat fall to very low levels—5 percent or below. Studies have shown that very low body fat in women can contribute to amenorrhea, or a disruption of the menstrual cycle. Female athletes may also experience weaker bones and flagging energy when body fat is too low.

CR practitioners naturally have lower body fat simply because they consume fewer calories. There is no need to try to reduce body fat levels further.

CR LOWERS LEVELS OF GROWTH STIMULATORS

Think of aging as a wheel spinning faster or slower depending on your rate of aging. As we've shown, too much glucose or insulin makes the wheel accelerate. The same goes for two growth stimulators: growth hormone and IGF-I (Insulin-Like Growth Factor). These work to produce changes in cells that lead to growth, which, as we've pointed out, is necessary when you are developing but can be damaging as you age. Fascinating studies by researchers at the National Institute of Aging and Southern Illinois University School of Medicine have linked decreased growth hormone levels to longer life span in mice—a life extension of up to 65 percent! Calorie restriction leads to lower glucose, insulin, growth hormone, and IGF-I and to the activation of SIRT1—all of which makes the aging wheel spin in slow motion.

EXCESS PROTEIN INCREASES IGF-I

Many studies of growth regulation in adults and children show that protein intake increases IGF-I levels—independent of calories. Research at Harvard University has shown that higher levels of IGF-I deactivate the longevity gene, SIRT1 (Cohen, 2004). And that's not all: more circulating IGF-I increases the incidence of cancer and the probability that existing cancers will grow to advanced stages (see page 111 in Chapter 7, "Cancer Protection").

We do not recommend combining CR with protein restriction, but keeping protein intake down to the DRI of 0.8 gram of protein per kilogram (0.36 gram per pound) of body weight is good advice. This translates to 43 grams for a woman who aims for a weight of 120 pounds and 56 grams for a man whose weight goal is 154 pounds. Remember: your number depends on your desired weight.

You may be familiar with the RDA (Recommended Daily Allowance) of nutrients. It was developed in the 1940s to protect populations of people from deficiency diseases. People have used the RDAs to try to optimize their nutrition. The U.S. government is building better tools for this purpose. DRI, a major revision of our nutrient and energy standards, is in development to replace the RDA, as we've known it. DRI—a generic term for several types of advisory reference values, one of which, ironically, is the RDA—is detailed in the glossary.

Another important factor to consider is protein absorbability. A standard evaluation of how well your protein is being absorbed and utilized within your body is the Protein Digestibility Corrected Amino Acid Score (PDCAAS), developed by the U.S. Food and Drug Administration and the United Nations agencies: the Food and Agricultural Organization and the World Health Organization. Because of the correlation between protein and accelerated aging, *The CR Way* includes dietary protein sources that are lower on the absorbability chart, such as beans and grains. The table shows a comparison of PDCAAS for some common proteins.

PROTEIN ABSORBABILITY

Whey	1.34*
Milk	1.21*
Brewer's yeast	**
Nonfat kefir	**
Nonfat yogurt	**
Egg white	1.18*
Beef	0.92
Soy	0.91
Kidney beans	0.68
Rye	0.68
Whole wheat	0.54
Lentils	0.52
Peanuts	0.52
Seitan	0.25

* On a strict scale, the maximum PDCAA score is 1.00 or 100%. To show the relative protein absorbability of foods at the top of the list we've included numbers from subsequent research. See the glossary.

** Official tests of these foods have not been reported yet. We include them here because in unpublished studies moderate amounts of these foods repeatedly produced significantly higher IGF-I readings.

CR PREVENTS CELL LOSS

As one ages, the body's ability to produce new cells decreases. As cells die, the inability of the body to replace them is thought by some to be at the root of aging—and of several age-related diseases. For example, researchers at Duke University found that older mice were unable to produce new cells that repair arteries, thereby causing atherosclerosis, the artery-blocking disease. Proving the point—when the old mice were injected with cells from younger animals, their repair processes immediately functioned normally.

Much research has been done on mice over the decades, showing that calorie restriction preserves their ability, as they age, to reproduce cells at youthful levels.

Does CR preserve the ability to reproduce cells at youthful levels in humans? Thanks to a collaboration between the Calorie Restriction Society and scientists at Washington University, led by Assistant Professor Luigi Fontana, M.D., Ph.D., we may soon know more about CR effects in humans. Dramatic results of CR's ability to prevent atherosclerosis in humans have been shown in a breakthrough study (Fontana, 2004). Plaque accumulation was found to be 40 percent lower in the arteries of the CR group versus the controls.

ARTERY WALL THICKNESS

AVERAGE WESTERN DIET	CALORIE RESTRICTED
0.7–0.9 mm	0.4–0.6 mm

Measuring the thickness of the carotid artery in the neck, an indicator of plaque buildup, can help predict coronary artery disease. The thicker the inner and middle layers, measured in millimeters, the thicker the artery walls and the greater the chance of atherosclerosis.

REJUVENATING BRAIN CELLS

Like the mythological Greek god Zeus, granting the mortal Tithonus eternal life but not eternal youth, it would be a cruel joke to slow the body's aging process without including the mind.

Some of the most exciting research today shows calorie restriction, rejuvenating nerve cells. This would increase the brain's capability for repair and cognition. Dr. Mark Mattson, renowned scientist and fellow CR practitioner, conducted research into CR's ability to rejuvenate new cells. His data suggest that CR is instrumental in 1) increasing the number of newly generated brain cells and 2) along with physical and mental activity possibly reducing the incidence and severity of human neuro-degenerative disorders.

Applying Dr. Mattson's research by practicing CR has produced measurable cognitive benefits—better long- and short-term memories, and sharper awareness in everything we do. By incorporating cognitive testing into your CR lifestyle through brain games, you will realize remarkable cognitive improvement. Learning to speak another language or to play a musical instrument has a good reputation for brain training. Measuring the results is easier, though, with mental proficiency exercises.

CANCER PROTECTION: OUT WITH THE OLD CELLS, IN WITH THE NEW

Disposing of malfunctioning cells through programmed cell death—which increases with age—is an important physiological process that helps maintain healthy cells.

Imagine a snake shedding its skin. The old, dead cells are sloughed off, and what emerges is a sleek, healthy, glistening creature: nature's own facelift. In tissues that are rapidly dividing—like skin, for example—CR increases the rate of this cell turnover, perhaps improving the health of the skin by hastening the death of dysfunctional cells.

Normally the body senses which cells are unhealthy and kills them before they have a chance to create dangerous mutations. As we get older, elimination of bad cells becomes less efficient. CR prevents this age-related decline in efficiency by increasing the rate of cell disposal of precancerous cells, which may be one of the ways CR protects against cancer, according to research by Dr. Stephen Spindler, one of the world's leading calorie restriction scientists.

Other leaders in this field, Drs. Haim Cohen and David Sinclair, proposed in a 2004 study that CR maintains physiological function by activating our hero, SIRT1, which protects necessary cells from dying off, thereby promoting the long-term survival of important, irreplaceable cells.

CR DECREASES INFLAMMATION

When most people think of inflammation they think of swelling, redness, and often pain. While not all inflammation is bad—it plays a vital role in the healing of tissue and immune system defenses—it is associated with many age-related diseases, such as arthritis and atherosclerosis. Some cancers and cardiovascular diseases are now also thought to be inflammation-related.

Being overweight fuels inflammatory processes because fat cells secrete chemicals that promote inflammation. Excess weight contributes to metabolic syndrome, which increases an individual's risk of coronary heart disease and other diseases related to plaque buildup in artery walls such as stroke, as well as Type II diabetes. CR reduces excess weight, thereby contributing to a reduction in inflammation.

Keep in mind that calorie restriction "thins the blood," that is, it reduces platelet adhesiveness, thus decreasing the potential for dangerous blood clots and the number of white blood cells—two essential components necessary to a successful immune response to inflammation. While these biological actions are thought to be beneficial, that does not mean that calorie restriction should be combined with multiple medications or supplements that have similar effects. Aspirin and fish oil, for example, also reduce platelet adhesiveness.

That's why we recommend forming a relationship with one or more doctors whom you trust and who will work with you. Aspirin is enormously beneficial in reducing inflammation in people at cardiovascular risk. However, since calorie restriction is already a serious intervention that reduces inflammation, you should always check with your doctor before adding aspirin or any other anti-inflammatory.

CR PRESERVES YOUTHFUL PHYSIOLOGY

Multiple choice: To preserve your youthful level of a vital hormone you:

A. Take lots of it.

B. Take herbs and other substances that provoke its secretion "naturally."

C. Understimulate it—causing the body to become more efficient in producing the hormone.

If you chose C, you selected one of the most beneficial ways to really intervene in the aging process.

Too much of a good thing can be harmful. Always keep *The CR Way* mantra in mind: *Less is more*. Indeed, we know that when the levels of many hormones are lower than usual, our cells increase the number of active receptors for those hormones, triggering an increase in our ability to use them.

We've already described the importance of limiting the secretion of growth-related hormones. This does not mean that you will lose the ability to produce these hormones, but rather, if you stick with CR for the long term, you have good chances of preserving the ability to produce these and other hormones and retain your body's sensitivity to use them into advanced age.

All of the biological benefits provided by CR work together to build your youthful physiology. By reducing your calorie intake, you will trigger hormesis and likely activate SIRT1 and other longevity genes. You will preserve your ability to do things like maintain a more youthful weight, have a more youthful heart, have a more youthful complexion. You may even get a better night's sleep by maintaining your ability to secrete melatonin, which helps regulate wake/sleep cycles.

With an understanding of the basics of *The CR Way*, you can easily adapt it to your own personal goals and lifestyle, whether you wade in slowly with a 5 percent to 10 percent calorie reduction or commit to a more serious 10 percent to 20 percent reduction. Whatever you decide, the science of CR will help you achieve a longer, healthier life.

2

EAT TO LIVE

Most Americans live to eat rather than eat to live, engaging in a love/hate relationship with food: love to eat, hate the results of overeating. Because eating is such an integral part of life, we often don't think about it unless we're planning to go on a diet. But how you incorporate food into your life—not just how *much* you eat, but what, when, and even how you eat—has a great impact on your health. With CR, limiting calories is the first step on *The CR Way* to longer, healthier life.

Before you embark on the CR lifestyle, first take a good look at the way you live. Like most of us, you probably have a fairly predictable lifestyle, maybe a little change thrown in now and then to mix things up. But for the most part, you have your own routine.

The CR Way can be adapted to fit any lifestyle because you are in charge of how much or how little you wish to reduce your caloric intake. The health benefits kick in with calorie reduction of as little as 5 percent, with benefits increasing as you further restrict and adhere to the overall plan. The choice is yours.

In order to get a better insight into your current lifestyle, use this simple **Healthy Lifestyle Gauge**. Rank each of the answers from 1 to 4, with 1 as most likely and 4 as farthest from the truth.

It's fair to assign a ranking to more than one answer. Once you have a sense of where you are, you can better plan where you want to be.

And be honest—you may know what the "right" answer is, but if it doesn't reflect your lifestyle, you won't benefit from selecting it.

FOOD

1. Which of these do you eat most?
      (a) All kinds of vegetables
      (b) Fish or poultry
      (c) Grilled food
      (d) Sugary desserts

2. When you want a snack, you reach for
      (a) Salty snacks
      (b) Raw carrot sticks
      (c) Chocolate chip cookies
      (d) A dish of blueberries

EATING HABITS

3. You generally eat
      (a) Right before bed
      (b) Several small meals
      (c) Early in the day
      (d) No breakfast, big dinner

4. You view food as
      (a) A security blanket
      (b) Fuel to keep your body running
      (c) Anything that's easy to swallow
      (d) A pleasure to be savored

5. You generally
    (a) Feel content enough that you don't think about food
    (b) Allow yourself to get hungry in anticipation of a meal
    (c) Always keep some food handy in case you get hungry
    (d) Eat until you are too full to eat anymore

ACTIVITY

6. You exercise moderately
    (a) More than 6 times per week
    (b) 3 to 5 times per week
    (c) Rarely if ever
    (d) Less than twice a week

7. Your preferred activity
    (a) Watching sports on television
    (b) Playing a sport
    (c) Taking a long hike in the woods
    (d) Stretching exercises only

8. You feel
    (a) You could stand to lose a few pounds
    (b) Heavy and self-conscious about your weight
    (c) Underweight and weak
    (d) Comfortable with your weight

MOOD

9. You feel
    (a) A slight energy lull in the middle of the afternoon
    (b) Cranky when you are hungry
    (c) Tired during the day and sleepless at night
    (d) Alert and competent throughout the day

10. You consider yourself
    (a) An optimist
    (b) A pessimist

SCORING: The following answer key will give you your score. Add together the numbers that correspond with your answers and see below.

1. a=1; b=2; c=3; d=3
2. a=3; b=2; c=4; d=1
3. a=4; b=2; c=1; d=3
4. a=4; b=2; c=4; d=1
5. a=1; b=2; c=3; d=4
6. a=1; b=1; c=4; d=3
7. a=4; b=1; c=1; d=3
8. a=2; b=4; c=3; d=1
9. a=2; b=3; c=4; d=1
10. a=1; b=2

10–16: Congratulations! You are already well on your way to a long, healthy life. *The CR Way* will enhance your focus on health and should be easy and comfortable to follow.

17–24: You have a healthy outlook and are headed in the right direction. You will find *The CR Way* to be an exciting and very feasible choice.

25–30: There are areas in which you can improve the quality and outlook of your lifestyle. *The CR Way* can help bring things into balance, and a moderate program may be a good place to start.

30–38: A life check is in order—you are allowing yourself to be controlled rather than taking control of yourself. *The CR Way* will be a challenge, but the results will be astonishing. Begin slowly, making incremental changes, and soon enough you will be pleasantly surprised to see and feel an entirely new you.

Whatever your score, by checking out the healthfulness of your own lifestyle, you have taken the first step toward a healthier, happier, and possibly longer life.

FOOD

Food fuels the body, and it also plays another significant role in our lives. Breaking bread together has long been a symbol of unity and friendship. Many will recall with pleasure those long, leisurely Sunday dinners with the relatives or the celebrations that weren't complete without rows of food-laden tables. Or perhaps you deny yourself food in order to lose weight and by doing so, mealtime becomes something to dread, food becomes the enemy.

How you view food will go a long way toward your success on *The CR Way*. By recognizing the nutritional value of the foods you choose—the caliber of fuel you feed your engine—you will learn to get the most nutrition from each calorie you eat. And on *The CR Way*, you'll find that nutrient-dense food is so delicious and satisfying that your relationship with food will become a happy means to achieving your goals, and not the focal point of your life.

The plan is not about denial but about choices. Making the healthiest choices to fuel your body while at the same time slowing down the aging process is the ultimate goal. The point is, you are eating for optimum health. Because the CR practitioner eats less, the effect of what you do eat becomes magnified.

What to Eat

Although based on calorie restriction science, *The CR Way* also emphasizes combining nutrients in the right way to trigger the longevity genes that exist in all of us. Research from Johns Hopkins, showing that low levels of fasting blood sugar may help activate the longevity gene SIRT1, means that a person on *The CR Way* limits both calories and glucose.

Not only the calories you consume but also the foods you choose determine the benefits you can achieve on *The CR Way*. Just as you want to pack as much nutrition into each calorie consumed, you want to know each calorie's effect—whether from carbohydrates, protein, or fats—on your glucose levels.

Carbs and Glucose

The total amount of carbohydrate and its absorbability are prime determinants of a food's effect on circulating glucose.

For example, broccoli has so little available carbohydrate that 100 grams would have a negligible impact on glucose levels, while the easily absorbable starch in 100 grams of white potatoes would send your glucose soaring.

Carbohydrates have the most impact on your glucose levels and are listed on what is called the Glycemic Index (GI), which ranks carbohydrates according to their effect on blood glucose levels. The higher the GI ranking in foods like white bread, sugary cereals, and many processed foods, the more they will elevate your blood sugar. Many vegetables and legumes have lower GI rankings. Fats and many protein sources have minimal effect on glucose levels and do not have GI rankings: no carbs—no GI. Carbohydrates that digest rapidly rank higher with a low absorption rate. Those foods that rank low on the GI, by definition, generally result in lower circulating glucose levels and thus less demand for insulin.

Glycemic Load

Your body's response to glucose in food depends not only on the carb availability of the food you eat, but how much. This is called the Glycemic Load (GL), first calculated by researchers at Harvard School of Public Health in 1997.

To determine the GL of a food, use this formula:

$$GL = GI/100 \times net\ carbs$$

(Net carbs are total carbohydrates minus the dietary fiber.)

GI rankings, which have been calculated by measuring glucose levels in blood samples from test subjects who have eaten various foods, can be found on a number of Web sites, including www.glycemicindex.com, run by the University of Sydney, Australia, where much of the research is done, or on www.mendosa.com, an excellent site for diabetics run by the renowned diabetes journalist David Mendosa.

The importance of measuring your glucose is covered in Chapter 4. It can be easy to do with a simple glucose meter like those used by diabetics.

Following is a list of the most common foods you'll enjoy on *The CR Way*. These are foods that are free of any serious impact on your blood sugar.

NO- OR LOW-CARB FOODS

VEGETABLES

Arugula

Beans, green, cooked

Beet greens, cooked

Bok choy, cooked

Broccoli, cooked

Brussels sprouts, cooked

Cabbage, cooked

Cauliflower, cooked

Celery root (celeriac,
   celery knob), cooked

Chard, Swiss, cooked

Collards, cooked

Cucumber

Dandelion greens, cooked

Eggplant, cooked

Kale, cooked

Mushrooms, cooked

Mustard greens, cooked

Onions, all types, cooked

Parsley

Peppers, bell—green,
   red, yellow, purple—cooked

Radicchio

Radishes, cooked

Rhubarb, cooked

Spinach, cooked

Squash, summer, cooked

Squash, zucchini, cooked

Tomatoes, stewed

Turnip greens, cooked

Watercress

FRUIT

Avocados

Cranberries (unsweetened)

Raspberries

Strawberries

FATS

Grapeseed oil

Olive oil

NUTS

Almonds

Hazelnuts

Pecans

(*table continued*)

Pistachios

Walnuts

(*table continued*)
EGGS
Eggs, chicken, poached

FISH
Salmon, Alaskan, wild caught, packed in water with no salt added
Sardines, packed in water

Although your glucose levels will likely be very healthy with these food choices, the way some foods are prepared will have an impact on your blood sugar. Puréed blueberries, for example, can elevate glucose (think smoothies). Overcooking many foods, such as lentils and beets, can also raise their glycemic impact.

When Low-Carb Foods Affect Glucose

If you have diabetes, even 1 gram of carbohydrate can raise glucose levels by as much as 5 mg/dl. Thus, a serving of 100 grams of strawberries, which has almost 5 grams of available carbohydrate, would raise glucose levels by about 25 mg/dl.

Foods that we often choose for our daily meals are ranked low to moderate on the Glycemic Index and include:

FOOD	GLYCEMIC INDEX
Barley	25
Lentils	28
Strawberries	40
Sweet potatoes	61

THE CR WAY CHECKLIST

On *The CR Way*, keep in mind—

- To restrict calories *The CR Way*, eat nutrient-dense food or food that has a specific functional benefit. See Chapter 9, "Foods to Choose," for more suggestions.
- To focus on eating foods that have low to moderate Glycemic Index rankings.
- To help foods retain their low to moderate glycemic effect by cooking them as little as possible. Keep vegetable boiling or blanching time to a minimum. Strain the vegetables from their broth to help keep them al dente. You can also plunge them in cold water to stop their cooking. Sprinkle them with lemon juice to prevent oxidation—especially sweet potatoes and beets.
- To limit total protein intake to around 45 to 60 grams per day for men and 40 to 50 grams a day for women. Using beans and grains as your major sources of protein will help you achieve this. Too much protein has been linked to increased cancer and accelerated aging. (See p. 16 for specifics.)
- To avoid added hormones and nonorganic fertilizers and pesticides by eating organic food whenever possible. Many of these unwanted additives are linked to cancer and birth defects.
- To make food intake heart-friendly by including some healthy fat source like walnuts or olive oil with every meal or snack. Healthy fat actually lowers the "bad" LDL cholesterol and triglycerides—both associated with increased risk of heart disease. Since fats can become carcinogenic when heated, always add them after cooking to avoid making them dangerous food sources.

You can see that *The CR Way* is loaded with vegetables, fruits, nuts, and legumes—all important to any healthful diet. While these are certainly not the only foods you'll find on *The CR Way*, the preceding lists offer you an idea of the kinds of healthful foods that will become a part of your new lifestyle.

What to Drink

Contrary to what many people believe, drinking liquids of any kind while eating will dilute important stomach acids needed for proper digestion. Don't drink liquids with your meal, but rather, drink between meals to refresh and hydrate without interrupting your body's nutritional absorption.

Pure water, vegetable broth, and herbal teas like dandelion, rosemary, or burdock are the best beverages to nourish your body. Just as with food, CR seeks to limit the empty calories you consume when you drink. High-sugar/high-calorie soft drinks, powdered drink mixes, and sports drinks too often provide lots of calories and

---

Q. Can I drink alcohol on *The CR Way*?

A. Many alcoholic beverages are the epitome of empty calories, the opposite of *The CR Way*'s nutrient density. Besides, the apparent protection against coronary heart disease conferred by wine has been debunked: The often-reported protective effect of moderate alcohol consumption on coronary heart disease disappears when twenty-four-year follow-up is examined. Further, high alcohol consumption became associated with higher risk of death from cancer with longer follow-up.

(Nielsen, 2005)

send your blood sugar soaring, with no measurable nutrients—exactly the opposite of CR.

We avoid caffeinated beverages because of their many detrimental effects. Here are some of them:

- elevates blood sugar
- elevates blood fats
- increases blood pressure
- stimulates central nervous system (may cause one to override the body's call for rest)
- causes irregular heartbeat
- increases urinary calcium and magnesium losses (may impact on long-term bone health)
- increases stomach acid secretion (aggravates a stomach ulcer)
- causes tremors, irritability, and nervousness
- causes insomnia and disruption of sleep patterns
- causes anxiety and depression
- causes heightened symptoms of premenstrual syndrome (PMS)

Q. And what about diet soft drinks on *The CR Way*?

A. In this case, you'll have to read the label, though we don't know of any that we'd add to our Foods to Choose. For example, lots of noncola soft drinks have caffeine in them. Many also include food additives that may have unwelcome effects. We'd rather drink nonstimulative herbal teas.

OPTIMAL EATING HABITS

The foods you choose are important to maximizing the nutritional value of every calorie. How you eat your meals and when you eat them are equally important on *The CR Way*.

How to Eat

A universal tenet of healthful eating is to eat slowly. Our fast-paced world is not geared for this, unfortunately, and all too often we find ourselves grabbing a bite as we race to a meeting or wolfing down breakfast at the kitchen counter as we hurry the kids off to school.

Not only is this bad for your digestion and probably your caloric intake, it can also wreak havoc on the way your body is processing the food you are eating.

Imagine someone is throwing a baseball to you. If it were only one baseball you would catch it—preventing it from hitting and hurting you. But if many people throw baseballs to you all at once, you couldn't catch all of them and some would cause injury. The same is true of the way your body processes insulin and glucose. If you select low-GI foods and eat your meal slowly so that glucose comes into your bloodstream gradually, insulin will do a great job of processing it. If, on the other hand, you eat quickly and/or include lots of high-glycemic foods, insulin will not be able to process the glucose fast enough, and it will run rampant in your bloodstream. And on CR, you want to reach low glucose levels in order to activate your longevity genes.

In many cultures, meals are eaten in long, leisurely courses, prolonging the enjoyment of each bite. *The CR Way* encourages this approach to eating. By stretching out your meal as long as possible you savor every bite, enjoying its delectable taste, texture, and nuances of flavor without thinking of what you are going to eat next. This may be hard to do when you first try it. Most likely, it will take concentration at first. That's why we included a detailed description of "Savoring Meditation" in Chapter 4. The idea is to use meditation to remove psychological pressures from the eating experience and revel in the foods that nurture us. As we rework our neural pathways to peace and happiness, small amounts of food are greeted with joy and appreciation. Calorie restriction becomes a liberation from the focus on amount of food to enjoying the quality of the experience.

The longer you extend your meal, the better your glucose control, digestion, and overall enjoyment will be.

When to Eat

If you are accustomed to eating three meals a day, there is no reason to stop on *The CR Way*. Always remember: The focus of CR is to eat nutrient-dense food to maximize the nutritional value you get from every calorie you ingest. While you will reduce your caloric intake, you can plan your meals in any order or schedule that works for you. We recommend enjoying a larger meal early and gradually tapering off as the day progresses to allow your body as much time as possible to process and absorb your food before going to sleep. See Chapter 3, "CR As You Like It," to guide you.

Regardless of how early or late you finished eating the day before, the overnight period before breakfast will almost always be your longest time away from food. During this fasting period, your insulin is likely to fall to low levels. When you break your fast, you are asking your body to make a 180-degree reversal from this low insulin state to the normal range for processing food and keeping glucose low. You want to help ease your body back into this normal state. Otherwise you are likely not to have enough insulin to process the glucose, leading to a spike in the level of glucose in your blood. Insulin will often respond by spiking, too—the *sudden* need to process food having shocked your system into producing more than necessary.

Break your fast as gently as possible—with a tablespoon of lemon or lime juice in a cup of warm water. Both of these juices, as well as vinegar, fit into the category of acidic foods that are known to lower glucose levels.

How to Lower the Glycemic Effect
of a Food or Meal

To lower the glycemic effect of a meal or recipe, simply add vinegar or lemon or lime juice to dressings, marinades, or sauces, according to the *GI Newsletter* (free online subscription) from the University of Sidney.

The acidity in these foods slows stomach emptying. Digestion of the carbohydrate in the food is therefore slowed, and the final result is that blood glucose levels are significantly lower.

Lemon or lime juice has the additional benefit of balancing pH by keeping your system from being too acidic. This is counterintuitive but true: These fruits, which contain a fair amount of citric acid, have an overall alkaline effect on the body. Still another benefit that makes lemon or lime juice a perfect way to break a fast is that both help cleanse the liver of toxins—a good thing to do on a regular basis. The lemon juice in warm water needs only fifteen minutes to work its magic. Warm water facilitates digestion.

The next key to starting your day with great glucose control is knowing how to eat to provoke the most effective release of insulin. Awaken your insulin production in a multistep process by:

• USING YOUR SENSES—enjoying food goes beyond taste, incorporating all the senses in anticipation of a satisfying meal. Immediately after drinking the lemon juice, we recommend that you activate the "cephalic phase" of insulin release. It's a kind of mind-over-matter process that is thought to be provoked by the sight, smell, and taste of food (before any nutrient is absorbed). A great way to awaken your insulin release this way is with very sweet sugarless gum. By itself this phase has shown modest results, but combined with a "tease meal" it can lower glucose levels by as much as 50 percent and sometimes more!

• THE TEASE MEAL—after chewing the gum (for as long or as little as you like), eat a small tease meal that helps your body ease into insulin production. The tease meal should consist of a small amount of your favorite carbohydrate food. Foods that are high in fructose are not the best choice for your tease meals since fructose does not help stimulate insulin.

Here are a couple of our favorite combinations:

		CONVENTIONAL MEASURES	GRAM MEASURES
1)	Sweet potato	¼ cup (scant)	50 grams
	Walnut	2 halves	4 grams
	Lemon juice	1 teaspoon (scant)	4 grams, or to taste
	Ground ginger		Sprinkles, to taste
2)	Tomatoes, whole canned	⅓ cup	80 grams
	Sprouted-grain bread	1 slice	34 grams
	Very Veggie vegetable cocktail Organic, low sodium	½ cup	125 grams
	Olive oil	1 teaspoon (scant)	4 grams
	Lemon juice/lime juice/vinegar		To taste

As you can see, the tease meal is just that. A small amount of complex carbohydrate goes into the system and is quickly converted into glucose that teases insulin into production. For those who choose a less rigorous CR regimen, breaking your fast slowly to allow your body a chance to "warm up" to insulin production is still a good idea.

• ADD SOME FAT—fat is an important nuance. We're not talking about bacon strips or jelly donuts, but insulin production and its actions are enhanced by fat in the bloodstream. That's why we include some delicious, healthy fat sources like walnuts or olive oil in our tease meals. You may also want to take a fish oil capsule with your lemon juice. The addition of omega-3 fatty acids supplied by the fish oil can help increase the amount of HDL cholesterol, lower blood pressure, and contribute to insulin release for glucose processing.

- EXERCISE—after eating this small meal and waiting approximately 45 minutes, give yourself fifteen minutes of moderate exercise—for example, yoga, weight training, rowing, or walking. This also stimulates insulin production and helps your body quickly return your glucose levels to baseline—a signal that it's time to start the rest of the meal.

- ADD MEDITATION—day-to-day life is full of major and minor stressors. Whether you are watching stock market results, working against a tight deadline, or cheering on your child's basketball team in a close game, your body is confronted with emotional or other adrenaline-provoking situations every day. Including fifteen minutes or so of quiet time for meditation during your morning routine can help keep glucose low, as well as lower blood pressure and heart rate, reduce stress, and increase cognitive capabilities. You will find that meditating will make limiting calories in an intelligent, serene way much easier. Objective decisions about making the best food choices and eating your meals at a reasonable, leisurely pace will naturally follow.

- MULTICOURSE BREAKFAST—controlling high glucose to gain the best benefit from CR is like winning a battle. Smart armies sneak up on their enemy at night, catching them while they are asleep before they have a chance to fight back. The same is true for glucose and insulin. Awaken your insulin and have it ready before glucose has a chance to rush in. Then is the time to enjoy a larger meal, including some proteins, vegetables, and healthful fat—pick and choose among the many Foods to Choose in Chapter 9 and the delicious recipes in Chapter 10.

Here is a sample of the meals on a typical day on *The CR Way*.

 The following breakfast serves as a model meal and will appear several times to illustrate various aspects of *The CR Way*.*

Morning Tease Meal, 88 Calories

	CONVENTIONAL MEASURES	GRAMS	CALORIES
Sweet potato	¼ cup (rounded)	70	53
Olive oil	1 teaspoon (scant)	4	35

Breakfast Main Meal, 805 Calories

	CONVENTIONAL MEASURES	GRAMS	CALORIES
Lemon-Ginger Salmon	3½ ounces	100	147
Potluck Vegetable Soup			
(weight of vegetables)	1 cup (scant)	200	84
Savory Barley (enjoyably combined with salmon and/or soup)	1½ cups	375	324
The CR Way Dressing	3 tablespoons	21	84
Lentils and tomatoes	½ cup	120	102
Raspberries and	½ cup	120	51
walnuts	3 halves	6	39

* For recipes. see Chapter 10.

Lunch, * 654 Total Calories

Lunch contains fewer calories and can be eaten at your normal noontime lunch hour, or if you choose to eat two daily meals, this one can be timed later and combined with dinner.

	CONVENTIONAL MEASURES	GRAMS	CALORIES
Green Bean Gourmet			
Sandwich	1 serving	125	126
Basic Beets—lightly			
boiled medallions	½ cup	100	69
The CR Way Garnish	3 teaspoons	15	47
Berries and Wheat Berries	2 cups	460	412

If you choose to eat dinner, it should be smaller, again containing fewer calories than your earlier meals.

Dinner, * 233 Total calories

	CONVENTIONAL MEASURES	GRAMS	CALORIES
*Mushroom Magic Cancer-			
Fighting Soup	1 cup	229	118
Genesis sprouted-grain			
bread	1 slice	34	80
Olive oil	1 teaspoon	4	35

Total Daily calories, 1782

This calorie intake would be fine for a woman who normally eats 2000 calories a day and has chosen to reduce her daily calorie intake by 10 to 15 percent.

Finally, don't eat late in the evening. We're always surprised when

---

* For recipes. see Chapter 10.

people who strive to be healthy tell us that they eat late at night. Using glucose control tools such as moderate exercise before going to bed is not wise. Studies (Monteleone, 1990) show that exercise before sleep disrupts the body's nocturnal increase of plasma melatonin—making good sleep unlikely. Oftentimes, the body takes five or six hours or even more to digest a meal. That means that a late-night meal can still be with you when you wake up in the morning.

HOW MUCH EXERCISE?

Praise for athletic achievement is so prevalent that people tend to think of exercise as how much they can push themselves. "No pain, no gain," the popular battle cry, is one of the most misleading and dangerous slogans ever to hit the gym. The best way to use exercise for most of us is for nurturing—helping the body make the most of its ability to adapt and heal.

Exercise is definitely associated with positive psychology. The big question most people want to know is how much. Chapters 6 and 8 and the FAQ in Appendix D provide more detailed answers. Besides the well-known cardiovascular benefits of physical exertion, the most important reasons to include exercise on *The CR Way* are these:

- To protect against osteoporosis
- To help control glucose levels
- To make our bodies strong enough so we maintain our strength and flexibility as we get older
- For cardiovascular health
- For relationship nurturing—an evening walk together, talking over the day

You should do something every day that at least gets you moving and your heart pumping. Lifting heavy weights twice a week will aid in osteoporosis protection.

Fasting—the Natural "High"

Fasting has a long, rich history of providing both physical and spiritual benefits—and with good reason. Giving your body a break from food facilitates healing to begin at the cellular level—flushing toxins, eliminating dead and dying cells while cleansing, nourishing, and spurring the growth of new cells. The best part of fasting, however, is the natural "high" you get that may result from the brain's release of the antidepressant-like chemical known as Brain-Derived Neurotrophic Factor, or BDNF.

Whether or not you decide to fast every day, you should try it at least every now and then. A fast that is long enough—up to fifteen to seventeen hours with fasting glucose in the 80s or below—will be likely to allow you to enjoy the release of BDNF. No drugs are necessary for the astounding natural high one gets from fasting.

While fasting is not a requirement for getting benefits from *The CR Way*, it will certainly make a difference in your mood—possibly changing it from happy to exhilarated.

3

CR AS YOU LIKE IT

The CR Way puts the science of CR to work for you, empowering you with the tools to live better and happier now—along with the best chance to avoid disease and live longer.

To start your journey on *The CR Way*, all you need to do is:

- Reduce your total calorie intake to between 5 percent and 20 percent, below normal for a person of your age, sex, height, and activity level. **To determine what your normal calorie intake should be, use the helpful chart provided below from the Health and Human Services/USDA Dietary Guidelines for Americans, 2005.**

- Control your fasting blood glucose to levels between 70 mg/dl and 90 mg/dl

- Keep your daily protein intake moderate (See page 16 for specifics.)

ESTIMATED CALORIE REQUIREMENTS

ACTIVITY LEVEL

Gender	Age (years)	Sedentary	Moderately Active	Active
Child	2–3	1,000	1,000–1,400	1,000–1,400
Female	4–8	1,200	1,400–1,600	1,400–1,800
	9–13	1,600	1,600–2,000	1,800–2,200
	14–18	1,800	2,000	2,400
	19–30	2,000	2,000–2,200	2,400
	31–50	1,800	2,000	2,200
	51+	**1,600**	**1,800**	**2,000–2,200**
Male	4–8	1,400	1,400–1,600	1,600–2,000
	9–13	1,800	1,800–2,200	2,000–2,600
	14–18	2,200	2,400–2,800	2,800–3,200
	19–30	2,400	2,600–2,800	3,000
	31–50	2,200	2,400–2,600	2,800–3,000
	51+	**2,000**	**2,200–2,400**	**2,400–2,800**

These levels are based on Estimated Energy Requirements (EER) from the Institute of Medicine Dietary Reference Intakes macronutrients report, 2002, calculated by gender, age, and activity level for reference-sized individuals. "Reference size," as determined by IOM, is based on median height and weight for ages up to age 18 years of age and median height and weight for that height to give a BMI of 21.5 for adult females and 22.5 for adult males.

Each of the following suggestions offers different benefits depending on your personal choices, needs, and goals. Fortunately, on *The CR Way*, you can choose a variation of the plan that fits your personality and lifestyle, changing and adapting it as you like.

5% CALORIE REDUCTION

A reduction of as little as 5 percent of your normal daily calorie intake will certainly improve your health.

At this level, you will cut about 100 calories from your daily intake if you are a woman of average size and activity, and approximately 125 calories if you're a man who is also of average size and activity.

A reduction of 5 percent may simply mean skipping your usual midday snack. *The CR Way* Foods to Choose are designed for maximum nutrition, and by following these suggestions, you'll find you are actually less hungry with fewer calories and your feelings of well-being and happiness will increase, knowing that you are eating healthful foods that nourish your body and spirit.

10% TO 15% CALORIE REDUCTION

A reduction of between 10 percent and 15 percent of your normal daily caloric intake will trigger hormesis, and your body will feel it. To enhance the CR effect of slowing cell proliferation, moderate your daily protein intake to the DRI of approximately 45 to 60 grams for men and 40 to 50 grams for women. (See page 16 for calculation factor.) You will begin to experience the longevity benefits of CR and decrease your likelihood of getting diseases like diabetes, cancer, and heart disease.

A 10 percent calorie reduction will mean shaving off approximately 200 calories per day for the average woman, 250 for the average man; 15 percent would reduce daily intake by 300 calories for the woman, 475 for the man.

Begin your breakfast slowly, as we've recommended, and make smart choices about the foods you choose for your meals. Your period of fasting will include your nightly sleep time. Still, you will want to "tease" your insulin back into production in the morning by savoring a nutritious, multicourse breakfast (see Chapter 2 for our breaking-your-fast recommendations).

While you may be consuming fewer calories than you are used to, consulting the Foods to Choose, Chapter 9, will help you make the best choices for your health. The recipes in Chapter 10 will ease your food preparation. You will find that with these new food choices and recipes, eating two or three meals a day will produce significant CR benefits. Try entering your food choices in nutrition-tracking software to know how much you are reducing your calories and what nutrition your diet is truly providing. With this knowledge, you will make informed choices about how to live *The CR Way*.

20% CALORIE REDUCTION

Comfortable now with your lower caloric intake, you are ready to further reduce calories by as much as 20 percent. We recommend that you limit your reduction to 20 percent so as to gain maximum longevity benefits while maintaining a lean but realistic body weight for your height and activity level.

On a 20 percent calorie reduction level, you will be cutting about 400 calories from your daily diet if you are a woman, 500 if you are a man. This is a completely manageable number as long as you continue to select foods like the nutrient-dense suggestions in Chapter 9.

You will find that occasional hunger is an integral part of *The CR Way*. The hunger sensation is not extreme and it can actually make you feel happy. Slight hunger is your body's signal that you are on the right track and doing what you've set out to do: eat less food than your body might crave so that you are more likely to attain your health and longevity goals. You will readily discover that slight hunger feels much better than the heavy, bloated sensation you used to get from overeating.

Be sure to keep your eye on the scale so you notice if you begin to lose more weight than is recommended for your height (see the BMI table in Chapter 7).

If improving cognition is an important goal for you, consider adding time away from food (see Chapter 4). This is most easily done by finishing your day's meals early enough to give you extra hours before breaking your fast the next morning. We usually get

Coping With Hunger

Hunger on *The CR Way can be welcomed* as your body's signal that you've achieved hormesis. Besides, the hunger hormone, ghrelin, actually *strengthens the heart!*

At the beginning of your *CR Way* journey, you may want to stave off hunger pangs. The following tips will help:

- Eat plenty of high-fiber foods that are low in calories but high in nutrients, like many vegetables and some fruits.
- Eat satisfying carbohydrates, but only those with low or medium Glycemic Index rankings, like those found in the Foods to Choose, Chapter 9.
- Add some delicious, healthful fat to your meal—besides being important nutritionally, fats slow your digestive system down, retaining the sensation of fullness longer.
- Plan your meals ahead of time. Don't wait until you are hungry to figure out what you're going to eat. If you do, you're likely to end up eating more than you intended.
- **Keep your "danger" foods out of the house, remembering that eating them is what keeps many people from reaching their goals.**

about sixteen hours away from food and find the cognitive and mood-enhancement effects very noticeable. While you can build in daily fasting at whatever amount of calorie reduction you are practicing, this may be a point when it feels quite natural.

Always plan to include some walking during your fasting period, aiming for glucose levels in the 80s or 70s during your fast. Take it slowly, not pushing beyond what feels comfortable. As your low-glucose fast extends to sixteen or more hours, your brain will turn

to ketones for fuel, and with that you may find your memory becoming sharper. Learning skills that you thought you had lost may
return. What's more, you may begin to feel happier as you experience a new brain chemistry that promotes optimism. If you include
some brain-training exercises in your plan, you may be delighted
with your newfound capabilities.

REMEMBER:

• Glucose control is an integral part of *The CR Way* and should be
practiced no matter which level you choose. This will further
decrease your chances of getting heart disease, diabetes, or cancer, and will very likely result in increased longevity benefits.
With the help of your trusty glucose meter, you can test your
glucose levels as described in Chapter 4. Adjusting your meals
and the way you prepare them will provide the benefits of glucose control, and you will probably find that you want to reduce
your caloric intake even further. The control of glucose levels
and getting no more than the DRI of protein (page 16), combined with calorie reduction, will provide excellent benefits.

• Practice meditation. As your body adjusts to lower caloric intake, you will find that meditation can help you increase all-
important rest and peace of mind. By incorporating meditation
into your plan, you will give a boost to the biological benefits
that living *The CR Way* produces—allowing contentment to replace thoughts of food and hunger.

You will probably discover that eating for the sake of eating just
doesn't feel right anymore. Unlike so many "diets," you are not de-
nying yourself the pleasures of delicious foods. While you may discover that the foods you choose have some new flavors, textures,

and nutrition than you've been used to, your priorities will change. You'll find yourself thinking more about how your new lifestyle contributes to your longevity and happiness than about what your next meal will be.

TIPS FOR DINING OUT

The CR Way as a lifestyle choice must fit into your existing life. You don't want to hide away in your kitchen, measuring each mouthful. You will want to enjoy sharing meals with friends, attending business lunches, dining at restaurants, entertaining at home—living your life to the fullest.

And then, of course, there are big family gatherings like Thanksgiving or birthday parties and general socializing with friends on a regular basis. How can you stick to your CR regimen? We enjoy dining out and do so within the parameters of our CR lifestyle. You can, too.

• Foods available on *The CR Way* are common, healthful foods found nearly everywhere. Special preparation requests can usually be made at restaurants.

• Let your dinner party host/hostess know about your CR regimen and offer to bring a prepared dish to share with the company.

• Reorganize your day to eat your biggest meal at dinnertime rather than breakfast or lunch, allowing you to enjoy a wider variety of foods while maintaining your calorie intake for the day.

• Invite friends or business associates to your home for dinner. So many of the recipes on *The CR Way* are delicious and "mainstream" enough to serve your guests. You may add foods for your guests that you might not eat, and you will make everyone feel welcome while sticking to your plan.

• An occasional splurge is all right. Now and then if you indulge in foods you might not generally eat on *The CR Way*, or perhaps eat more than you normally would, it's okay. Don't be too concerned. Go ahead and eat some mashed potatoes, but try not to heap them onto your plate. See if you can stick to poached salmon rather than grilled steak for your protein, and always think twice about the gravy. Ask for steamed vegetables, and why not share a dessert with a friend rather than eat it by yourself? What matters is that if you are doing CR most of the time, overall, your health will be better. Do remember, though, that occasional bingeing may be dangerous—especially for someone practicing CR for a long time. Your system isn't used to processing large amounts of food. Like everything we do on *The CR Way*, moderation is the key.

• Your family and close friends will be aware of your lifestyle choice and guess what: they won't care! People who care about you will be supportive of your choices and will gladly work with you to keep you on the right track.

People often exaggerate the importance of eating in *good* relationships at gatherings. In fact, whether or not you eat is not so much the point. How you treat other people with whom you share a meal is what matters. We treat others with kindness and thoughtfulness and try to see their best qualities—hoping to help them feel good about themselves. Believe us, at the end of the meal, if you have done just those things, you will have friends for life who won't be likely to say, well, gee, I don't know about those people—they didn't eat this or that.

Another thing that will happen almost spontaneously is that people will begin to want to know what it is that you are doing. Why aren't you looking any older? And you don't seem to get tired anymore. At that point it is likely that your friends may take more than a casual interest in your new lifestyle and think about trying it themselves.

PART II

BENEFITS TO THE BODY AND MIND

4

GLUCOSE CONTROL: THE SWEET SPOT IN LONGEVITY

Nutritionists, dieticians, dentists—even your mother—caution you to go easy on the sweets. Too much sugar can wreak havoc on your diet and your teeth, and it may even accelerate aging.

A vital key to the CR lifestyle is learning to control your glucose, just as you control your calories. One way to accomplish this is by managing your carbohydrates, the primary source of food that the body breaks down into glucose. And by controlling glucose, you'll contribute further to your overall longevity plan. (And your dentist will love you!)

GAUGING YOUR AGING

Wouldn't it be great if you had a way to gauge how well you are controlling aging? Measuring blood sugar levels may be helpful.

Hoping to slow down aging without knowing your glucose levels is like trying to drive a car without a steering wheel.

Major Types of Sugar

Glucose:
Most dietary carbohydrates contain glucose, either in starch and glycogen, or together with other sugars.

Fructose:
A simple sugar contained in honey, fruits, and some root vegetables. All fructose must be metabolized in the liver, while glucose can be processed by every cell in the body.

Galactose:
A sugar found in dairy products, beets, and gums

Sucrose:
Commonly called table sugar or saccharose

Lactose:
A sugar found in milk

Chances are you will have a wreck before you get where you want to go.

Begin with knowing what your glucose levels are—both when fasting and after a meal. It is not sufficient to know what your fasting glucose levels are from lab tests at your doctor's office. You need the practical knowledge of how your glucose levels react to how you live—the foods in your diet, meal timing, exercise, etc. To find that out, you should use a blood glucose meter, a simple device used by diabetics that can be found in most drugstores, surgical and medical supplies stores, or on the Internet.

People balk at the painful pricking of fingers that using a glucometer used to entail, but fortunately those days are over. Many glucose-testing systems are pain-free and easy to use. Glucose meters for use on the forearm and the thigh instead of the high-sensitivity fingertips are easily available. For a great list of glucose-testing options, consult Mendosa.com, an online diabetes resource.

Many meter producers will provide you with free starter kits that contain all the tools necessary to get started—glucose monitor, a few test strips, lancets, and instructions, etc. Buying the test strips regularly can be fairly expensive. But it's a small price to pay for the age-slowing insights provided.

Fasting Glucose Levels

Normal	Above Normal (Prediabetic)	High (Diabetic)	CR
Up to 100	100–126	126 or more	74–88*

Units: measured in milligrams per deciliter (mg/dl)

*Fontana L (2004)

Note: lower levels achieved by intense exercise do not extend life in lab animals.

Since the longest period of low glucose is likely to be overnight, testing your fasting glucose before eating anything in the morning is very informative. To have the best chance of keeping glucose at low, healthful levels, try the suggestions in this chapter about how to eat, exercise, and time your meals. You can test as little or as often as you like.

WHEN TO TEST

Use the glucose meter to test your glucose levels when you first get up. That number is your fasting glucose level, or **baseline,** the number your insulin-secreting cells will likely try to return you to after you have finished eating. When you first begin CR, your levels will probably be in the 80 to 100 range, the average fasting glucose level for most people. Your goal will be to reduce it to the CR levels of 74–88.

When Glucose Goes Too Low

When fasting glucose levels suddenly go much lower than people are used to, they may experience negative effects, such as confusion, dizziness, irritability, or depression—even passing out. Like any other aspect of *The CR Way*—moderation is the key. When lower fasting glucose is a goal, do it gradually—aiming for a maximum lowering of 10 mg/dl (as measured on your blood glucose monitor) over a two- to three-day period. Once you achieve it, go no lower for a few days to allow your body to adjust.

If you do experience symptoms of low glucose levels by going too low too fast, eat some easily digested carbohydrate, e.g., puréed sweet potato—easily available as baby food, which you could consider having on hand.

Next, try testing after a meal. Depending on your food choices, you may be surprised to see how quickly the foods with high amounts of easily digestible carbohydrates make a difference in your glucose levels—usually taking only fifteen to twenty minutes to show up.

Once you are comfortable checking your glucose levels, you can decide when to test new food choices and combinations. Knowing your blood glucose levels will help you make decisions about your food choices.

At the beginning, however, in order to understand fully the impact that glucose has on your ability to function optimally and possibly to trigger your longevity genes, we suggest using the glucose meter at twenty-minute intervals after a meal until the glucose levels return back to your baseline number. When you try this for the first time, the results may be quite shocking. Foods that you thought were "healthful" may produce alarmingly high glucose spikes. And you have reason to be concerned: Sudden glucose spikes can be dangerous and are linked to cardiovascular risk.

Q. Do I have to test my glucose every morning before I eat?

A. No, you don't have to test every day. However, when just beginning *The CR Way*, testing provides an excellent gauge to see how you are doing and make sure you're on the right track.

The CR Way steps to great glucose control provide glucose-control goals for the model meal outlined in Chapter 2—incorporating a "tease meal" about an hour before your main meal. Note that altogether, this is almost a nine hundred-calorie meal, which might be expected to produce a very large glucose influx. Yet the glucose-control methods described here will keep glucose rises confined to a small range. These results are consistent with studies, showing that use of a small tease meal before a larger meal produces superb glucose control.

THE CR WAY TO GREAT GLUCOSE CONTROL

BREAKFAST:

Step 1

Measure fasting glucose (your "baseline")—**Your goal: 70 to 85 mg/dl**

Step 2

For the initial glucose-lowering effect, start your food intake with lemon juice in water—warming the water first to make it "lemon tea" if you like.

Lemon juice	1 tablespoon	(7 gram)
Water	1 cup	

Activate cephalic insulin production by enjoying sweet sugarless gum

Step 3

Enjoy a small tease meal of mainly moderate-GI carbohydrate foods mixed with some high quality fat to help activate insulin production:

 Sample Tease Meal, *88 Calories:*

	CONVENTIONAL MEASURES	GRAM MEASURES	CALORIES
Sweet potato	¼ cup	70	53
Olive oil	1 teaspoon	4	36

Step 4

Incorporate fifteen minutes or longer of moderate exercise like yoga, walking, or weightlifting—followed by Centering Meditation (page 84).

Step 5

Measure your glucose after you finish your exercise. **Your goal:** return close to baseline before starting your main meal.

Step 6

Breakfast Main Meal, 805 Calories (For recipes, see Chapter 10)

	CONVENTIONAL MEASURES	GRAMS	CALORIES
Lemon-Ginger Salmon	3½ ounces	100	147
Potluck Vegetable Soup (weight of vegetables)	1 cup (scant)	200	84
Savory Barley (*enjoyably combined with salmon and/or soup) (includes mushrooms and onions*)	1½ cups	375	324
The CR Way Garnish	3 tablespoons	21	84
Lentils and tomatoes	½ cup	120	102
Raspberries and	½ cup	120	51
walnuts	3 halves	6	39

Step 7

Measure the glycemic effect of your main meal starting twenty to thirty minutes after you finish eating. **Your goal:** postprandial (after the meal) glucose levels to remain within 10 to 20 mg/dl above your baseline.

Step 8

Use the blood glucose meter to see how long it takes your blood sugar to return to baseline after your meal. **Your goal:** To keep glucose low, let **glucose levels return close to baseline** *before eating anything else.*

WHAT IF YOUR FASTING GLUCOSE LEVEL IS TOO HIGH?

You've followed *The CR Way* closely and have tried everything, but still have stubbornly high fasting glucose levels. Before you panic and self-diagnose Type II diabetes, relax and consider that your body constantly adjusts to meet what it believes to be the norm for you. Your "norm" would be the baseline number you saw when you first tested your morning glucose level, probably in the 80-to-100 range. Remember, on *The CR Way*, we are seeking levels closer to the 70-to-85 range. More specifically, the cells that secrete insulin—your pancreatic beta cells, or b-cells—tend to remember your fasting level of glucose. Like an alarm clock that buzzes at the time to which it's been set, the b-cells return your body to the glucose levels set by your eating habits.

Our experience confirms that the glucose baseline is not set in stone. Rather, it is constantly being reset, depending on meal timing, food choices, and length of fast. Resetting your glucose to a lower fasting level is easy. Here are some resetting suggestions:

1 Finish your last meal of the day as early as possible, making sure to eat a complex-carbohydrate meal consisting of low-GI carbs and a high-quality fat source. Eat as small a meal as you can get by on, but enough to stimulate insulin production.

High-Quality Fat?

Not all fat is bad. Adding some high-quality fat sources like olive oil, fish oil, or walnuts to a meal can improve cardiovascular health.

2 Plan your meal so you have plenty of time to a) take a forty-five-minute or longer walk after eating, and b) two or more hours for the food to be digested before going to bed.

3 Measure your glucose to see the effects before and after the walk. Most likely the glucose will be lowered—perhaps even reset—to the new baseline you are aiming for. If not, continue walking until your reading gets to within 10 points or so of your goal.

Glucose Is Glucose

Some health enthusiasts do not take the glycemic rate of foods into account when choosing foods for their diet. They seem to think that as long as a food is classified as a "health food" it is okay. That is hardly the case, as raw versus processed sugar, honey, liquefied fruits, pureed high glycemic vegetables are not good for you just because some extra vitamins or antioxidants are thrown in. The effect will be largely the same: high glucose, more AGE (Advanced Glycation Endproducts, see page 68), more triglycerides, etc.—and, very likely, quiescent longevity genes.

When you wake up the next morning, you may be pleasantly surprised to discover that your fasting glucose is already reset. Whether it is or not, follow the glucose-control protocol as previously outlined, being careful to choose foods that have low GI rankings. If possible, add moderate exercise sometime after your main meal, with the goal of returning your glucose to fasting levels before you eat anything else. Continue to follow this routine until your fasting glucose regularly tests at healthy levels.

IMPORTANT: COOKING METHOD MATTERS

Already your glucose monitor may have tipped you off to the fact that so-called "low glycemic" foods can produce unpleasantly high glucose levels. This is often related to how the food is prepared. Just as puréeing can greatly increase the rate of glucose absorption from many fruits and vegetables into the bloodstream, so too can the amount of heat and length of cooking time. For example, lentils are a wonderful bean and when lightly cooked do indeed have a moderate glycemic effect. They develop a much higher GI if cooked until they are mushy. Differences in preparation methods and the resulting glycemic effect are very pronounced with some vegetables. Beets, for example, lightly steamed or blanched and eaten in reasonable amounts, have a moderate glycemic effect. Eat them mashed—particularly a lot of them—and watch your glucose levels soar, likely turning off your longevity genes.

You will want food choices and meals to raise your glucose levels as little as possible, and as you follow *The CR Way*, those levels will naturally drop along with calorie intake. Every reduction that you achieve by food selections and timing is terrific.

Keep track of your glucose levels with the blood glucose meter, comparing these variables to see what works for you. Then you can decide if and how you want to work toward your goal: no more than 20 points above your starting point or baseline.

Following is an example of how even a small amount of puréed sweet potato affects glucose levels over a two-hour period.

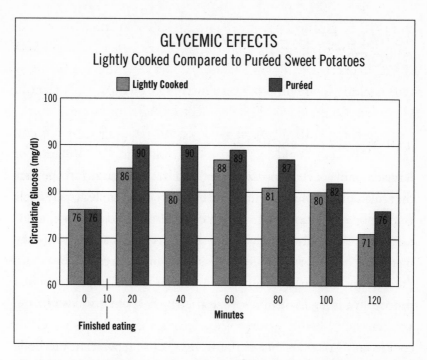

GLYCEMIC EFFECTS
Lightly Cooked Compared to Puréed Sweet Potatoes

The effect of food preparation on glucose levels: In unpublished research, the glycemic effects of puréeing versus lightly cooking a small amount, 90 grams (3.2 ounces), of sweet potato were compared. To keep the sweet potato tests heart healthy, two grams of olive oil were added to each test meal.

The sweet potatoes were eaten first thing in the morning to break a fasting period of seventeen hours. After fasting, when insulin levels are low, even a small amount of carbohydrate can make a big impact, as this seventy-five-calorie example shows. The insulin available right after fasting was no match for the puréed sweet potatoes. They drove glucose levels higher than the lightly cooked preparation, and glucose stayed high for forty minutes.

In contrast, available insulin easily dispensed with the slow carbohydrate absorption of the lightly cooked potato. Glucose levels never got above 87 and they didn't stay there very long. What's more, insulin production had plenty of time to manage the slow glucose influx from the lightly cooked potatoes, efficiently sending circulating glucose to seven percent below baseline within the two-hour-and-twenty-minute test period.

BEWARE OF **AGE** (ADVANCED GLYCATION ENDPRODUCTS)

Overcooking food will produce something called AGE, Advanced Glycation Endproducts. Development of AGE occurs when proteins combine with sugars or fats; so, too much glucose running rampant in your bloodstream also contributes to the formation of large amounts of AGE. AGE is nothing but biological garbage that prevents optimal functioning of your molecules. AGE accumulates in the body over time and is linked to disease and functional deterioration, especially in tissues like the heart and brain. It would be one thing if this waste could be cleared from your system, but that's not so easy. Reversing AGE accumulation is still an experimental process. Your goal is to minimize the AGE content in everything you eat.

Helen Vlassara is one of the world's leading AGE researchers. Her studies have shown the link between AGE and increased risk of age-related diseases and have also identified the kinds of foods that have an impact on your AGE levels. One of her lab's studies found that the food we eat can be a significant source of AGE. This may be a chronic risk factor for cardiovascular and kidney damage.

Vlassara and her research group have concluded that heating foods causes AGE formation. The three aspects of food preparation that increase AGE content in foods are higher temperatures, the length of cooking, and the absence of moisture. So how you cook your food is critical in minimizing AGE. The higher the cooking temperature, the longer the cooking time, and the less water used, the more AGE is produced.

The following cooking methods are listed in decreasing order of AGE production:

Broiling (225° C)
Frying (177° C)
Roasting (177° C)
Boiling (100° C)

Roasting is lower in AGE generation because it uses so much more moisture than frying does.

Vlassara and her team note that the highest AGE content is found in foods of the fat group as well as meat and meat substitutes. Spreads including butter, processed cream cheese, margarine and mayonnaise contain the highest level of AGE. Animal products high in proteins and fats like meat and cheese also have high AGE content, especially industrially processed foods—frankfurters, bacon, and powdered egg whites, for example.

The carbohydrate group contains the lowest AGE. If you follow the food recommendations of *The CR Way* you will be getting little AGE.

AGE CONTENT OF SELECTED FOODS
THE LOWER THE NUMBER—THE BETTER

FOOD ITEMS	SERVING SIZES	AGE UNITS*
Vegetable soup, Homemade	1 cup	3
Tea	1 cup	5
Yogurt (low fat)	1 cup	8
Cantaloupe	3.5 oz	9
Apple	3.5 oz (less than ½ cup)	13
Egg white boiled × 10 min	30 gm. (small)	13

(*continued*)

(*continued*)

Green beans, canned	3.5 oz	18
Sweet potato, roasted	3.5 oz	72
Egg yolk boiled × 10 min	15 gm (small)	182
Avocados	30 gm (2 tablespoons heaping)	473
Cheese American processed	30 g	2,603
Frankfurter, broiled	90 gm (one)	10,443

*AGE units are milligrams of N-carboxymethyllysine, a well known advanced glycation endproduct.

HOW TO AVOID AGE

- Never eat foods that have been cooked for a long time.
- Always cook with moisture (water, broth).
- Steam, poach, or boil foods.
- Avoid all high-heat cooking methods.
- Never cook longer than necessary to kill microbes and make the food digestible. Cooking al dente is best for avoiding AGE, and it makes foods chewy and delectable, too.
- Remember that foods continue to cook after they are removed from the heat, because of their internal temperature. Take advantage of that when preparing foods like sweet potatoes or beets, for which you can reduce the cooking time and more easily enjoy them cooked to perfection.
- Never cook fats—add them after cooking food.
- Never eat browned, grilled, or fried foods. The skin on browned or fried foods is full of AGEs.

- Never add sugar, fructose, or galactose to any food.
- Do not microwave anything except water.
- Reheat previously cooked foods in a tempered glass pitcher or ceramic bowl in a heated waterbath on the stove. It's a double boiler concept: the bowl is put into a pan of water on low heat.

Possible AGE Inhibitor?

Benfotiamine is a vitamin B-1 derivative that is available without pre-scription. Several studies have confirmed that benfotiamine can reduce AGE formation in humans.

(Stirban, 2006)

FRUCTOSE: FRIEND OR FOE?

Fruits and vegetables are dietary staples, among the most highly recommended foods for proper nutrition. The fructose found in fruits and some vegetables may also seem like a good way to control glucose. On the surface it seems attractive, since it produces a very low glycemic reaction, compared to table sugar.

But fructose is no bargain: Several studies have shown that fructose has a stronger tendency than glucose to form AGEs, which, as we know, can contribute to age-related disease. Therefore, we recommend limiting your fructose consumption to no more than 10 grams/day.

Fructose Content* of Common Fruits

	Per 100 gm of edible portion
Prune (dried)	12.49
Grape	6.9
Pear	6.60
Apple	6
Kiwifruit	4.4
Banana	4.85
Blackberry	3.4
Blueberry	3.28
Strawberry	2.5
Orange	2.4
Cantaloupe	1.87
Grapefruit	1.7
Raspberry	1.7

Based on USDA Standard Reference Data as supplied by NutriBase

GLUCOSE CONTROL THROUGH SAVORING MEDITATION

One of the most important aspects of glucose control is to learn to eat slowly, giving insulin time to manage the carbohydrates that are processed by digestion. Managing your glucose takes time and patience, but it should never become a burden. *The CR Way* is about much more than limiting calories or glucose: The point is always to live a healthier, happier, and longer life.

Meditation is incorporated into the CR lifestyle to assist in dealing with the challenges your dietary changes may present. A big benefit of meditation is to help you be in the moment—not thinking about what you are going to do, but about what you are experiencing right now. That is especially important for enjoying food—making it easy to reduce calories.

Savoring Meditation

Even if you have no difficulty in limiting calories, taking the time to heighten the joy of your eating experience can be achieved with Savoring Meditation—a contemplative enjoyment of very small portions of food in which you savor every bite for its taste, texture, and smell.

Breaking your morning fast is an ideal time to experience Savoring Meditation, an opportunity to take full pleasure in your first meal of a new day.

Blueberries are good for practicing Savoring Meditation because of their subtle texture, taste, and smell, as well as their beneficial effects, which may include better memory and possibly even life extension.

With comfort in mind, you will find it helpful to wake up the mind. Stand and raise yourself up all the way on your toes and reach for the sky—as you do so, take a deep breath in. Now exhale as you descend slowly and come to a relaxed, erect position.

Now, try it again and as you come down let out a big sigh—just as if all your frustration, sadness, and anything that makes you unhappy could be let go in one big *ah-h-h*.

Repeat for a third time.

Now shake your arms vigorously for about thirty seconds.

When you are ready, sit down and find a comfortable seated posture, back straight, preferably sitting away from the back of the chair. Now gently close your eyes. This will help you focus on the wonderful sensations that you will experience.

With your eyes closed, direct your attention to your feet. Feel well grounded so that all parts of your foot—toes, sole, and heel— are firmly connected to the floor. Take a moment to focus on each toe. How does each one feel? Is it relaxed? What do the joints feel like? Let each toe feel long and rest naturally on the floor. You may discover a great deal of tension in your feet; your toes may feel tight or cramped. Let them be warm and limber, just like noodles in a soup.

When you are ready, let the relaxed feeling in your feet emanate through your entire body, first, through your legs and eventually to your buttocks. Let the muscles of your buttocks relax—each gluteal muscle should exert equal pressure on the chair. Let your spine lengthen and widen with dignity so that you come into a posture that feels wonderful and is a joy to maintain.

Now, you may be wondering what to do with your hands. Hand positions vary from one meditation practice to another. We recommend holding your hands on your knees with the palms up, open to the air. Or if it feels more natural, rest them gently on the chair beside your legs.

As you open your hands to the air, notice that they are sensitive to the way the air feels—whether it is warm or cold, whether there is a breeze or not.

And when you are ready, extend the awareness of the air touching your hands: Expand it so that the air touching every part of your body cradles and comforts you.

And now with your whole body feeling wonderfully relaxed and long and wide and in touch with the air around you, bring your attention to your breath. Unless you have a cold, breathe through your nose to feel the sensation of air moving through your nostrils. And if it feels natural, carry your awareness of the incoming air all the way down into your lungs and even down to your abdomen as it gently expands and contracts with every breath. As you breathe, notice on the in-breath that the body seems to pause naturally, and on the out-breath there is also a natural pause.

Don't worry if your mind wanders. That is natural and it happens to everyone. If you experience it, don't be hard on yourself. Just gently and intentionally bring your mind back to your breath.

Also notice that as you breathe in and out, your palms and fingers may actually feel the ever-so-subtle movement of air that your breathing creates. Imagine yourself in a garden where you see grass and leaves gently swaying in a soft breeze.

Now expand your image of the garden. Perhaps you have a garden or a picture in your mind of how the garden that you love would look. Are flowers of many colors growing there? Is green grass between the flower beds? Are some of the flowers tall and others close to the ground?

As you walk in your garden, the earth feels slightly soft to your feet. You feel the sun warming your back and arms and hands, and as you look up to the sky it is blue with wispy white clouds. Occasionally you hear the mystical and mellow cooing from a dove that is just out of sight.

In your garden is a chair where you decide to sit in the tall, dignified manner you have adopted. See yourself sitting in your garden.

As you sit down, you notice that on the table beside you there is a gift. Your heightened sense of smell lets you know that some food has been left beside you, and as you pay close attention to what's there you actually smell the sublime scent of blueberries, and think what it would be like to break your fast by eating just one of them. First you could take it in your spoon and bring it to your nose, inhaling deeply to thoroughly enjoy the smell. Then you could touch it to your lips and consider how to get the blueberry from your lips to your tongue. When you do take the blueberry in your mouth, you let it roll around on your tongue. Can you feel the texture of the blueberry? Is the skin smooth or does it have slight indentations?

As the picture of eating becomes more vivid in your mind's eye, you may begin to activate insulin production so that when you eat a full meal later, insulin will be ready to effectively mop up circulating glucose.

Now open your eyes and take a blueberry from the bowl beside you and actually bring it under your nose and smell it—can you tell how it's going to taste just by the aroma?

Close your eyes again and as you put the blueberry into your mouth, pretend you are part of a film shown in slow motion. Before you bite into the berry—roll it around on your tongue. Can you feel its round shape with your tongue? Can you already taste it—even without biting into it?

And when you are ready, slowly bite the berry. What teeth do you chew it with? Does it break into pieces? Can you feel the juicy, tender inside? And how does it taste? Can you savor the distinctive blueberry flavor on your tongue—where? In the center, at the back of the tongue, or perhaps all over? As you swallow it, perhaps you will continue to taste it even after it has passed into your stomach.

This time take two blueberries with your spoon—and a walnut. Again take time to hold them in your mouth for a moment. What is the walnut shaped like? Can you feel how it contrasts with the blueberry? Where does the walnut stimulate the taste sensation? On your tongue? On your palate? Is it also in your cheeks and in your nose? How do the blueberries taste this time? Is the flavor more intense? Or perhaps the foods have melded together, creating a new distinct flavor. And notice, if you will, that you can even savor the blueberry and walnut all the way up in your brain, as many parts of your body are activated by the blueberry experience.

Once you have finished the blueberries, put your eating utensils down, close your eyes, and return to your breath for a moment.

Imagine how wonderful it would be to eat a whole meal this way. How will you eat your next meal? Will it be at top speed in front of a computer, or will you slow it down, savoring each moment and each bite—increasing your ability to experience your long and happy CR life?

Now, as you end your practice, open your eyes when you are

ready and get up slowly, treating yourself to a gentle return to the marvelous day you are experiencing.

SPECIAL BENEFITS OF GREAT GLUCOSE CONTROL

As you gain control over glucose levels, you begin to notice how they affect your ability to function. You can use this knowledge to plan glucose levels that enhance your ability to excel at various tasks. For example, low glucose levels are known to produce a brain chemistry that increases cognitive capabilities and makes a person feel more optimistic. Memory and reaction time also increase when glucose levels are in the 90 mg/dl to 100 mg/dl range.

A rule of thumb we have learned over time is that sudden large influxes of glucose can interrupt concentration and make it difficult to think clearly. Needless to say, we avoid meals and food combinations that spike our glucose.

Both restricting calories and controlling glucose are vital keys to *The CR Way*. They naturally go together: One must pay attention not only to the calorie intake, but also to the nutrient density of the foods the calories come from and how the nutrients in those foods will interact with the body's chemistry.

It can feel like a biology lesson and at times, it is. But to live a longer, happier, more productive life, we need to know how our bodies work in order to help them function to their maximum potential.

5

MIND MATTERS

We've all experienced it at one time or another: You meet an acquaintance on the street and suddenly can't remember his name, or worse, call him by the wrong name. You can't remember where you put your keys or what you did with the grocery list that you need for the market; you forget to return your movie rentals.

These cognitive hiccups seem to become more frequent as you age. But memory loss and cognitive dysfunction are not inevitable, and *The CR Way* can help you maintain and sharpen your mind.

Imagine how happy you would be if you could find a prescription that magically rejuvenates your brain cells, firing up your neural pathways and allowing you to think clearly and absorb and process information quickly and easily. By following *The CR Way*, you will bathe your brain in chemicals that help form new neural pathways. This formula creates a mood of happiness and exhilaration and improves relationships—making it easier to do things *you* want to do.

To get started, here is *The CR Way* Rx for a better brain:

• BURN KETONES—an efficient, fat-burning source of energy that is triggered by low glucose.

• INCREASE LEARNING CAPABILITIES—CR increases the secretion of learning-enhancing substances.

• PRACTICE MEDITATION—meditation enhances your CR experience and produces physical changes that benefit brain function.

• EAT BRAIN FOOD—staples of *The CR Way* to a better brain.

• SLEEP—nothing like a good night's sleep for better thinking— *The CR Way* improves the length and quality of your sleep.

• TRAIN YOUR BRAIN—sharpen your mind by practicing brain exercises.

BURN KETONES

Although the brain weighs only three pounds, or approximately 2 percent of body weight, it uses 20 percent of the body's circulating glucose, our major source of energy. So when we lower our glucose levels, we trigger an elaborate energy-backup system that produces an alternate form of energy—known as ketones—to sustain energy flow when glucose levels fall.

Ketones, according to researchers like Dr. Richard Veech of the NIH (National Institutes of Health), are not only an alternate energy source, but a superior one because they increase the efficiency of your metabolism while decreasing the production of damaging "free radicals," which are by-products of normal metabolism. "Magic," he calls them. Dr. Veech has studied the use of ketones to treat neurological disorders such as Alzheimer's and Parkinson's diseases. Other recent studies have documented the antioxidant effects of ketones and their potential role in protecting the cells' energy producers—the mitochondria. In essence, ketones produce significant brain-protective improvements. This is why we plan our *CR Way* to activate ketone production.

In diabetes, ketones are often a warning sign of low insulin and high blood sugar.

But calorie restrictors are intentionally reducing blood sugar to a level low enough to activate ketones for energy.

DAILY LIMITED FASTING

Whether your CR diet induces ketones has a lot to do with your method of calorie restriction. Many calorie restrictors eat several small meals throughout the day. Others split their daily caloric intake between two large meals with space in between. These methods of CR are unlikely to induce much ketone production because glucose levels never get low enough to activate ketones.

We call our method of CR "**Daily Limited Fasting.**" For us, this means a large CR meal in the morning for breakfast and then a smaller CR lunch. And that's it. Stopping eating around 1:00 p.m. or so, we fast until the next day, fifteen to seventeen hours. Much of this time our glucose levels are in the 80s or below—the low range necessary to produce ketones. Eating even just a little during the fasting period will cancel the ketone production.

More About Ketones

Q.: What if I don't want to fast so long? Can I still get some benefit?

A.: The key to these ketone benefits is maintaining low glucose long enough for blood ketone levels to reach the 0.3–0.5 mmol range, which is at the high end of normal for a healthy person with low glucose.

The ketone body for calorie restrictors to measure is b-hydroxybutyrate in blood or urine.

b-hydroxybutyrate (blood levels)	Reference range	Status
	<0.6 mmol (10.7 mg/dl)	Normal
	0.3–0.6 (5.3–10.7)	Ketogenic CR
	>0.6–1.5 (7.2–27)	Risk level for diabetics
	>1.5	Ketoacidosis

Studies have shown that the lower glucose availability causes positive adaptations—forcing cells to use glucose more efficiently. Meanwhile, CR also preserves neurotransmitter levels, which are vital to the cells' ability to exchange information.

Our Daily Limited Fasting regimen is based on research by Dr. Mark Mattson and his colleagues at the Laboratory of Neurosciences, at the National Institute of Aging, in 2003. They found that time away from food was even more valuable than calorie restriction for increasing beneficial brain chemistry.

Like the hormesis triggered by restricting calories, the body responds to the stress of periodic fasting in a similar way, triggering protective proteins in the brain and stimulating regeneration of brain cells. This is a very important finding for anyone who wants to increase personal brainpower.

The CR Way to Ketones

A ketogenic diet, often used in controlling epileptic seizures, is usually described as a meal plan that emphasizes large amounts of protein and fat—not the best way to practice CR.

Daily Limited Fasting, offered on *The CR Way*, also produces ketones but through a healthful complex-carbohydrate diet.

Don't feel you need to go to an extreme level of fasting to achieve the kinds of benefits we get from ketone production. You are already fasting during the eight hours you sleep at night. Adding another few hours to your fast won't feel the least bit extreme! The secret to ketone production is keeping glucose low during the fasting period—not the specific number of hours spent fasting.

INCREASE LEARNING CAPABILITIES

Like the hormesis that produces runner's high, CR creates a stress-induced release of brain-nurturing chemicals that help the brain form new neurons, which make learning and retaining information easier. One of the chemicals that helps generate new neurons is the same one we talked about on page 43 as giving the natural high to people who fast—Brain-Derived Neurotrophic Factor, or BDNF.

Similar to the endorphin rush in runner's high that causes a feeling of euphoria, studies confirm the positive mood effect of BDNF. Low levels of BDNF correlate with depression and many antidepressant medications combat clinical depression by increasing BDNF levels in the brain. CR does this naturally!

PRACTICE MEDITATION

Meditation is an integral part of *The CR Way*. Besides the calming and centering that make it easier to do CR, meditation can actually create beneficial changes in the brain structure. Meditating increases the thickness of the brain's cortex in areas involved in attention and sensory processing.

Centering Meditation

We recommend doing the Centering Meditation in the morning when the beneficial brain chemistry provoked by CR is likely to be at its height. First, break your fast—perhaps with lemon juice in warm water. Then enjoy your tease meal (Chapter 2) and whatever form of moderate exercise you have decided to do for your morning glucose-lowering routine.

After exercise, your mind should feel awake and ready to meditate. Find a quiet place where you won't be disturbed. Some prefer to sit comfortably. Lately, we find that standing can be slightly more effective. Then close your eyes and begin by being aware of your breathing. Just pretend you are watching your breathing like you might watch a leaf, moving about in a gentle breeze. Then pick a word or phrase that has meaning for you.

Silently repeat your chosen word or phrase each time you exhale. When stray thoughts appear, be easy on yourself—this happens to everyone. Just gently escort your mind back to watching the breath and repeating your phrase. Meditating for fifteen minutes or more is a good goal.

When you want to stop, slowly open your eyes and enjoy the peace and calm, which can last for hours. Just as sleep recharges your brain, meditation helps focus it, letting you use your newfound energy for positive, productive efforts all day long.

Meditation has been proven to make measurable differences in thinking capabilities. In a 2005 study of mental acuity, for example, researchers found that subjects who meditated before taking a test to evaluate response time showed superior performance.

EAT BRAIN FOOD

Remember how your mother used to tell you to eat fish, "it's brain food?" Once again, Mother knows best.

Fish Oil

Omega-3 fatty acids, are commonly found in fish, particularly fatty fish like salmon, as well as some plants, nuts, and seeds. The omega-3 fatty acids have been so well documented to improve cardiovascular health that doctors often prescribe them for their heart patients. Their role in brain health is also important. The brain is 60 percent fat, so it must have sources of fat to function. Two members of the omega-3 family, EPA (eicosapentaenoic acid) and DHA (docosahexaenoic acid), are especially important in the brain: EPA helps to increase blood flow while DHA helps to transmit nerve impulses. Addition of EPA and DHA to the diet has been documented to improve cognitive performance in children.

On a calorie restriction diet, eating enough food to supply adequate levels of omega-3 fatty acids would be very difficult indeed, because CR'ed bodies are busy burning some of their fatty-acid intake for fuel. For this reason, we recommend taking a fish oil supplement. When we began to use fish oil supplements, we experienced a noticeable increase in mental capabilities, as well as a more optimistic feeling overall.

In fact, Dr. Andrew Stoll, director of the Psychopharmacology Research Laboratory at McLean Hospital in Boston, has found that the EPA in omega-3 directly enhances mood, and he has successfully used it to treat bipolar disorder, a disease that includes bouts of severe depression.

Fish Oil Side Effects

Whenever you take supplements or medication, consider the side effects. People who are taking a blood-thinning medication should be aware that fish oil also thins the blood. Other side effects may include:

- Fishy odor on the breath
- Upset stomach

How to Select the Right Fish Oil

LOOK FOR:
- High amounts of omega-3: 800 to 1100 mg. per day
- Clear, bright yellow caplets for better digestion
- Molecular distillation, separating oil from toxins for a purer supplement IF the source fish are up the food chain, e.g., cod, but not plankton-eating sardines, mackerel, and anchovies
- Produced with nitrogen to prevent oxidation and rancidity

(continued)

(continued)
- Listed source of fish oil, including fish type and location. (Cold-water, small, oily fish like sardines or anchovies are preferred because they are less likely to have pollutants.)

IT SHOULD NOT HAVE:
- Strong, fishy odor which indicates rancidity
- More than 50 mg of omega-6, 500 mg. (0.5 gm) of omega-9, or 500 mg of saturated fat
- Vitamin E, which can prevent proper breakdown of fats

FOR IMPROVED MOOD:
- Higher ratio of EPA to DHA (7 EPA to 1 DHA)

FOR LOWERING BLOOD PRESSURE:
- More balanced ratio EPA to DHA (3 to 2)

Of equal importance is the amount you take: Never take more than what is recommended on the label unless advised by a doctor to do so. Laboratories have documented that excessive intake of fish oil can result in high amounts of lipid peroxides, which are associated with cell membrane damage and accelerated aging.

Protein

Foods that are high in protein increase the brain-alertness chemicals dopamine and epinephrine. Research shows that when the brain produces more dopamine and epinephrine, brain power is heightened and the ability to concentrate and react quickly is increased.

But wait—didn't we say earlier that protein can increase age-accelerating hormones? Yes: That is why many alertness-provoking foods like brewer's yeast, whey, egg whites, soy protein, and low-fat meats like chicken or turkey are usually off-limits for us—because they are so high in protein. We make exceptions for special occasions.

We do get some of our protein from small servings of salmon twice a week and one whole egg per week. The rest of the time we use bean and grain combinations for protein sources. This gives us enough protein—50 to 60 gm/day—to provide the alertness chemicals we need, while keeping age-accelerating hormones like IGF-I low.

Cholesterol for Cognition

Cholesterol has gotten a bad rap over the years, and deservedly so when talking about heart health. But it does have a positive impact on the brain.

In the famous Framingham heart study, which recruited more than five thousand people from Framingham, Massachusetts, and has followed them for fifty years to study heart disease, researchers found that total cholesterol strongly correlated with cognitive performance. It was found that lower naturally occurring total cholesterol levels are associated with poorer performance on cognitive measures such as abstract reasoning, attention/concentration, word fluency, and executive functioning.

Those who scored higher on cognition tests had cholesterol levels above 200 mg/dl—a level that would be considered to be a risk factor for cardiovascular disease. We don't try for anything nearly that high. But we do try to keep cholesterol from falling below the 110 to 120 range, healthy for good artery and heart function while still affording some of the cognition benefits.

Cholesterol that's too low

If you are zealous about seeing how low your cholesterol can drop on a CR diet and you allow your cholesterol levels to plunge to below

100, BEWARE! Cholesterol is not only important for cognition, but also for mental health: low cholesterol has a strong association with depression and suicide.

Further linking cholesterol to mental state, higher cholesterol levels help increase serotonin, the calming chemical that is so important for relaxation. Many experts have suggested that low cholesterol can cause dieters to break their diet, binge, eat sweets, etc., because of a need for more serotonin in their brains.

SLEEP

Long, deep, restful sleep is an important part of any lifestyle. Study after study has confirmed that length and depth of sleep affect both cognitive skills and length of life.

Many people report moments of problem-solving insight after a good night's sleep. Makes sense—during sleep, the brain processes new memories and solves problems.

Researchers at the University of Pennsylvania have confirmed that lack of sleep impairs mental performance. Study participants were divided into four groups that received eight, six, or four hours of sleep per day for fourteen days, or no sleep for three days. To our surprise, researchers found that sleeping less than six hours a night for many nights in a row was as bad for mental performance as going without sleep at all for a few days. Participants were evaluated by a testing regimen that included reaction time, ability to think clearly, and simple memory tasks.

Subjects were not allowed to use caffeine or any other stimulants. Thus, the results show what really happens to mental acuity when people do not override their natural state with artificial stimulation.

Sleep also affects length of life, regardless of health status. Research has shown a link between poor sleep and early death. A University of Pittsburgh School of Medicine study found that sleep disruption, such as prolonged bouts of wakefulness at night—thirty minutes or longer—can double the risk of death in healthy older adults.

The CR Way Improves Sleep Quality and Length

CR increases the quality and length of sleep, quite possibly because, as shown in animal studies (Roth, 2001), CR slows the age-related decline in the hormone melatonin, which regulates sleep/wake cycles.

In addition, CR seems to enhance the body's own natural tendency to lower temperature in preparation for sleep. Perhaps that's why when we enhance that effect by keeping the temperature in the bedroom low, we find it easier to fall asleep and to sleep longer.

CR Reduces Body Temperature

The slower heart rate, decreased metabolic rate, and lower circulating glucose produced by CR combine to reduce average body temperature. This is consistent with studies showing that lower body temperature is associated with longer life.

Interestingly, studies have shown that lower body temperature contributes to longer life, but whether it is due to reduced oxidation or hormonal stress, the exact mechanism is still to be discovered. Since lower body temperature is thought to be an important CR longevity effect, we avoid excess heat—taking shorter, cooler showers, avoiding use of electric blankets, and the like, that counter CR's natural age-slowing cooling effect.

Although CR preserves the sleep-inducing secretion of melatonin, great sleep is not guaranteed. With all of life's distractions, try to develop a sleep strategy that helps you to sleep longer and better like the ones offered in the following table.

SLEEP STRATEGIES

- Eat high-protein foods—such as beans or salmon, which activate brain-alertness chemicals—early in the day.
- Get out into the sunshine during the day—exposure to the sun sets your body clock to activate melatonin at night.
- Eat carbohydrate foods for your last meal of the day—carbohydrates produce the calming serotonin for relaxation.
- Turn the lights out at the same time every night to send a strong circadian signal to your body that it is time for sleep. You may want to meditate in the dark for a few minutes before going to bed.
- Listen to the same piece of relaxing music each night just before bed.
- Keep the bedroom as dark as possible.
- Eat the last meal of the day well before bedtime—never rely on a full stomach to put you to sleep.
- Never take a supplement or food or drink that is artificially stimulating (see Chapter 3, "Eat to Live," page 34).
- Keep your bedroom cool—somewhere in the low 60s F.
- Use an air purifier to keep the air you breathe refreshing, pure, and relaxing.
- Have some "white noise" in your bedroom to help tune out sounds that keep you awake or awaken you—use earplugs if sounds that disturb you are likely.
- Place a pillow under your knees when lying on your back to take the strain off your lower back.
- Use a "flattenable" pillow under your head so that the axis

from your hips along your spine to the top of your head
remains straight.

- If you sleep on your side, use a pillow thick enough to keep
  your head in perfect alignment with your spine.

Softness Meditation for Sleep

If you have trouble going to sleep or if you wake up and can't get
back to sleep, Softness Meditation can be a huge help. It also works
wonders for taking short daytime naps that rejuvenate brainpower.

Softness Meditation starts by concentrating on your hands. The
hands are wired with the most nerves of any area of the body, so
they will respond readily to signals from your brain.

Start with your dominant hand. Begin by concentrating on your
middle finger. Think of the first joint of your middle finger as
growing soft, long, and spongy. Use your imagination to match the
softness in your joint to the softness of your mattress, sofa or wher-
ever you choose to meditate. As you feel the softness and spongy
length come into the joint, carry it on to the next joint in your finger, feeling it grow just as long and soft as the previous joint. Finally, concentrate on the smallest joint of the finger until your
finger feels limp, like a wet noodle.

Notice that by doing this, you are distracting yourself from wor-
ries, hunger, or any other thoughts that may keep you awake. Once
you are satisfied with the soft feeling of your middle finger, continue the same procedure with your other fingers, progressively relaxing the joints in each of these fingers in exactly the same way.
Let your fingers carry the wonderful relaxed feeling they are enjoying into the palm of your hand and up to your wrist. Match the
feeling in your wrist to the soft feeling in your whole hand. As your
relaxation deepens, it may almost seem like you have gotten a shot
of a muscle relaxant in your hand. If you had a muscle pain somewhere in your body, you may have noticed by now that it has

significantly reduced. If by chance you have a pain in your arm or shoulder, start your softness meditation in the hand opposite to the pain, because it will be much easier to send a clear relaxation signal to your brain.

Now repeat the procedure finger by finger in your other hand. Just by deeply relaxing your two hands, you may already have drifted back to sleep. But in case you haven't, continue the wonderfully relaxed feeling in your hands all the way up your forearm into your elbows. Let your forearm grow long and spongy and the elbow joint grow soft. Continue to carry that feeling into your shoulders, stopping at each shoulder joint, then right up the often tense and tight muscles between your shoulder and neck. If any of these muscles becomes difficult to relax, refer back to your hand—making it so relaxed that the rest of your body cannot resist.

Let your neck be free and your spine feel longer and your back, wider. Your whole body should begin to feel just as soft as your mattress and pillow.

Let the relaxed feeling extend to your face. First let the muscles around one eye be soft. Connect the space between your eyes so it too feels very soft and supple. As your eyes and the space between your eyes become very soft, relax your eyebrows and your forehead to match. Let the relaxed feeling extend all the way down your scalp, tell your ears that they feel soft and the muscles around your mouth feel soft and relaxed, while your jaw just naturally feels loose and drops. As you practice Softness Meditation, you will begin to look younger as furrows in your face begin to fade, along with the mental anguish that put them there.

Now let the relaxed feeling extend all the way down, through each rib, so your chest naturally expands. You can pretend that the musculature between your shoulder and hip joint is completely loose. As your hips relax, continue to your knees, stopping to unwind any tension in these complex joints, leaving them just as relaxed as your finger joints. Continue "lengthening" the joints in your ankle and the long bones of the feet. Progressively relax the joint in each toe, matching the softness in your toe joints to the joints in your fingers. During this meditation you may actually find yourself drifting somewhere between sleep and wakefulness in a very blissfully relaxed state.

Once you master Softness Meditation, you will find it's not only useful for putting yourself back to sleep at night, but also to put yourself to sleep anytime you need a little rest to perform optimally. Rather than drinking coffee or taking stimulating supplements to stay alert for long workdays, the secret is as simple as developing the ability to take short catnaps if energy wanes—sometimes for only a few minutes.

Taking It Easy with Serotonin

Getting enough serotonin, the brain's calming chemical, is important for psychological health. Serotonin has a wide range of actions. It helps control mood, sleeping, waking, and temperature regulation. It also plays a role in blood pressure regulation.

Serotonin can also have a major impact on your diet. Some nutrition scientists cite low levels of serotonin as the primary reason people cannot stick with diets. Too much serotonin is associated with sluggishness and decreased sex drive.

Keeping the right balance of serotonin is an important part of *The CR Way* because it contributes to the feeling of satiety— making it easier to say those magic words to yourself or to others: "Thank you—I've had enough food." Serotonin, which is released in the brain after a carbohydrate meal, ushers in the calm, mellow feeling that is so important to mental health. It can also be used to relax in a tense situation. Performers, public speakers, athletes— anyone who is in a high-pressure situation—can use a serotonin-producing meal to bring about the calm that could make the difference between a good performance and a great one.

To Keep the Serotonin Flowing

- Eat carbs with moderate GI rankings, like sweet potatoes, to facilitate serotonin production in a healthful way. All it takes is a snack of two-thirds of a cup of sweet potatoes to produce the pleasant calming effect of serotonin forty-five minutes later. Add a little olive oil to make the snack heart-healthy. If you sense that your serotonin levels are low, eat more carbohydrates for your last meal of the day to help you prepare for sleep.

- Finish eating high-protein foods at least three hours before your carbohydrate, serotonin-provoking meal—the last meal of the day.

- Note that the serotonin-producing effect of carbohydrates works best on an empty stomach.

Tryptophan, the amino acid that produces serotonin in the brain, is found in protein sources like turkey and milk. **But don't be fooled—eating foods like these that are high in protein will *not* increase your serotonin!** Tryptophan is not absorbed well in the presence of other proteins. Neither does fruit work well as the carbohydrate source for triggering serotonin, because foods that are high in fructose do not spark the necessary chemistry to allow tryptophan to be properly absorbed. Your best bet for increasing serotonin through your diet is to eat complex carbohydrates with a moderate glycemic rating, such as sweet potatoes, stewed tomatoes, or sprouted-grain bread.

Train Your Brain

Just as you exercise your muscles with weights, yoga, and other tools, you can exercise your brain with a variety of cognition-improvement programs to take advantage of all the chemical enhancements produced by CR. We like to "train" our brains right at the end of our fast when brain-benefiting chemistries are likely to be at their peak.

Any cognition-improvement book will probably recommend learning new skills such as a foreign language or a musical instrument. Just make sure that you develop your new skill to the best of your ability. Don't try to take on too much all at once, but rather, practice a few fundamental cognitive tasks until you can perform them at a very high level. Consider the world's greatest classical musicians who retain their very fine motor skills to advanced ages. Most likely they have developed several key études to a very high level of proficiency that carries over into every piece they play. The same is true of developing a high level of cognitive skill on fundamental thinking tasks—it will carry over into everything you do.

Another tip: Set goals for yourself as a way to measure your increasing cognitive abilities. For example, if playing an instrument, master a particular piece of music and with each practice session, play that piece at a little higher standard of performance. Establishing a regularly achievable level of competency at a cognitive task provides a standard to measure against. That way when you decide to add something to your routine, like a new supplement or food, you will be able to assess objectively how it affects your cognitive skills.

Sequential processing is the ability to receive and utilize information in an orderly way. It is a vital aspect of memory and learning.

A very effective way to improve sequential processing is to use brain-training software. This will help you improve your thinking capabilities to very high levels and improve everything you do.

6

HEALTHY HEART

Recently, strong evidence has shown that the hearts of CR practitioners function like those of much younger people. In 2002, we worked with scientists at Washington University to help organize and participate in a human study where eighteen individuals who had been practicing CR for at least six years were compared to eighteen age-matched, healthy people on typical Western diets. Not only did the CR participants in the study achieve extraordinary results on a battery of tests that measure cardiovascular health, our group—with an average age of fifty—had blood pressure numbers equivalent to those of ten-year-olds!

Normal aging causes the heart to become less efficient in the way it pumps blood to the rest of the body. In the passive diastolic phase—the lower number on your blood pressure reading—the heart's left ventricle first fills up with blood to about 80 percent, and then the left atrium of the heart contracts to completely fill up the ventricle. As we get older, less blood gathers during this phase, so the atrium has to pump harder to fill the ventricle. On CR, our hearts were found to perform this task like those of people fifteen years younger. While very low blood pressure is good, evidence that our hearts were aging slower was the exciting finding.

BLOOD PRESSURE COMPARISON:
CALORIE RESTRICTORS, A CONTROL GROUP,
AND 10-YEAR-OLD CHILDREN

	CALORIE RESTRICTORS (Average age 50) (Fontana, 2006)	CONTROL SUBJECTS (Average age 50) (Fontana, 2006)	10-YEAR-OLD BOYS (NIH analysis, 2005)	10-YEAR-OLD GIRLS (NIH analysis, 2005)
Systolic BP	99.1	129.13	102	102
Diastolic BP	61.6	79.7	60	61

Another path to heart health is exercise, and the American Heart Association recommends thirty minutes of physical activity every day to help prevent cardiovascular disease. This approach to exercise is in keeping with *The CR Way*: moderation in everything. Interestingly, research has shown that intense, extensive exercise like that of endurance athletes has no more effect on maintaining healthy diastolic heart function than the activities of a control group of nonathletes. Maintaining a moderate exercise regimen is the key. Exercise and *The CR Way* are covered more extensively in Chapter 8: "Getting Started."

Heart Attack and Stroke

The calorie restriction studies at Washington University (Fontana, 2004) tested for any signs of atherosclerosis, the artery-clogging disease that leads to heart attack and stroke. The testing included an ultrasound scan of the carotid artery, the main artery that supplies the head and neck with blood. The thicker the walls of the artery, the more plaque, which is an indicator of heart disease and a precursor to heart attack. Reviewing the scans projected on a screen, researchers were amazed to see virtually no plaque accumulation on our artery walls.

Q. Doctors recommend an aspirin a day to help prevent heart attack. Can I still do this on CR?

A. Aspirin is enormously beneficial in reducing inflammation in people at cardiovascular risk. However, since calorie restriction is already a serious intervention that reduces inflammation, you should always check with your doctor before adding aspirin or any other anti-inflammatory medication.

CAN HUNGER STRENGTHEN THE HEART?

Because you are restricting calories on *The CR Way*, you are bound to feel hungry at some point during the day. But that's okay—in fact, it's better than okay. Some hunger feelings are extremely beneficial. During hormesis—the hunger hormone, ghrelin, is secreted by the stomach, making the heart adapt and begin to use fats much more efficiently for fuel. Studies have shown that ghrelin increases the heart's stroke volume—or the amount of blood pumped through the heart's left ventricle, which is an indicator of cardiac output—both in healthy volunteers and in chronic heart failure patients. Further, long-term administration of ghrelin as a medication improves heart function and reduces the weakness and fatigue associated with chronic heart failure.

That's why we aim to be slightly hungry sometime during the day. Usually these periods last only a few minutes. Rather than feeling weak or droopy when we are hungry, our bodies have adapted and we feel quite energetic. The occasional stomach growl doesn't automatically send us to the refrigerator for a snack, but rather, we greet the hunger with satisfaction, knowing that we've practiced our calorie restriction routine correctly.

Please understand, this is not a recommendation for extended hunger periods, malnutrition, or muscle wasting. Work with a doctor who checks you on a regular basis to make sure your practice produces positive results. Should you feel any continued muscular weakness or extended fatigue, simply eat a little more. So, no matter what your goals are, you are always listening to your body and using common sense to respond to warning signals.

FIBER FOR THE HEART

Fiber, carbohydrates that cannot be easily digested, is an important nutrient for lowering cholesterol levels and regulating digestion. On *The CR Way*, fiber plays a vital role in your daily diet, primarily because many of the foods that are best for human health—grains, vegetables, fruits, nuts, and seeds—are very high in fiber. The American Heart Association recommends including fiber in your diet every day, approximately 14 grams per 1,000 calories consumed. Because of the focus on grains and vegetables in *The CR Way* diet, calorie restrictors may often consume 70 grams to 80 grams of fiber per day or more.

Fiber is classified as soluble or insoluble, based on whether it dissolves in water. Fiber's solubility determines the nature of its beneficial effects on health.

Insoluble fiber, like that found in dark, leafy greens and many seeds and nuts, accelerates bowel motility and cleans your intestines as the stool passes through. This cleansing action may prevent cancer-causing substances from remaining too long in the intestine and it may improve the microbial balance of the gut (microbes feed on the fiber that we can't digest).

The water-soluble fiber in foods like barley, beans, and fruit not only helps reduce cholesterol, but at least one such type of fiber, beta glucan, found in oats, barley, some mushrooms and other

Garlic for the Heart

Garlic, a daily part of our CR diet, has been used as a blood thinner and anticoagulant to resolve blood clots and improve circulation. It has been shown to lower cholesterol while increasing the level of beneficial HDL (high-density lipoprotein), the so-called good cholesterol.

In addition, garlic compounds gently lower blood pressure by slowing the production of the body's own blood-pressure-raising hormones. At least seventeen clinical trials have shown that mild hypertension can be effectively managed with garlic.

foods, can be beneficial by reducing the LDL cholesterol that is strongly linked with heart disease. In fact, in a Harvard study of more than forty thousand male health professionals, researchers found that a high total dietary fiber intake showed a 40 percent lower risk of coronary heart disease, compared to a low fiber intake.

The scientific evidence backing heart-benefiting effects of fiber prompted the FDA (Food and Drug Administration) to allow health claims to be made on the labels of foods containing soluble fiber from whole oats (oat bran, oat flour, and rolled oats). The claim notes that foods that contain at least 0.75 gram of soluble fiber per serving in conjunction with a diet low in saturated fat and cholesterol may reduce the risk of heart disease.

Because dietary fiber is not readily absorbed, many CR practitioners subtract the fiber count from their total daily caloric intake to get a better understanding of and estimate of the calories their bodies will actually absorb.

Consider the contrast between a typical CR breakfast and a traditional American one:

THE CR WAY BREAKFAST

FIBER ANALYSIS

FOOD ITEM	SERVING SIZE	FIBER
Barley, pearled, cooked	1.3 cups	11 gm
Lentils, boiled	3.6 oz	7 gm
Very Veggie low-salt, organic vegetable cocktail	1 cup	2 gm
Strawberries, frozen, unsweetened	3.4 oz	1.5 gm
Blackberries, frozen, unsweetened	0.8 oz	1.2 gm
Tomato, Tuscan, canned	4.8 oz	1.1 gm
Mushroom, boiled	6.6 oz	0.9 gm
Walnuts	1.5 oz	0.6 gm
Onion, steamed	18 gm	0.3 gm
Lemon juice	18 gm	0.07 gm
		Total fiber: 27.15 gm

TYPICAL AMERICAN BREAKFAST

FIBER ANALYSIS

FOOD ITEM	SERVING SIZE	FIBER
Whole wheat bread	1 slice	1.932 gm
Orange juice	8 fl oz	0.130 gm
Bacon	2 slices	0.000 gm
Margarine	1 tbsp	0.000 gm
Egg, poached	3.3 oz	0.000 gm
		Total fiber: 2.06 gm

Too Much of a Good Thing?

Including enough *insoluble* fiber, from vegetables like spinach and cauliflower and other sources such as whole flax seed, in *The CR Way* diet is important because too much *soluble* fiber in some CR diets can actually slow bowel motility and negatively affect the microbial balance. We recommend a delicious solution by eating one or more servings each day of hulled barley (see glossary)—a great insoluble fiber source and hearty addition to soups. If reading this inspires you to increase your fiber intake, do it slowly. Increasing fiber suddenly can cause intestinal pains, gas, diarrhea, or constipation. And, as previously mentioned, don't drink liquids with your meal, but rather, between meals so as not to dilute stomach acids, which can, in turn, disrupt digestion.

Moving your bowels fully every day will prevent the toxic load produced by stool accumulation. Full bowel evacuation will help the whole digestive system optimally perform its vital role of digesting food and making nutrients usable by the body, which is especially important on a reduced-calorie diet.

What if your stools are too loose or you have problems with diarrhea? This may make you feel weak—robbing you of the energy and ultimately the robust feeling you can get from *The CR Way*.

Diarrhea or constipation problems can mean the microbial balance in your digestive system is unhealthy. Fortunately, probiotics are available. These supplements supply good bacteria that can help correct microbial imbalances. Because they are considered dietary supplements, they don't need FDA approval, but among the ones we've found success with are:

- *Lactobacillus GG*—especially good for diarrhea
- *L. acidophilus+L. casei*—capsules only
- *Bifidobacterium infantis* 35624

If you decide to try a probiotic, don't assume that taking lots more than the recommended amount is a good idea. The recommendations are based on research results. And just like any gut bacteria, even the good ones may cause gas and bloating in the beginning as your system adjusts to it. After about ten days, you will likely feel substantially better.

Make sure you take your probiotic well away from any spice like cinnamon or cayenne, any herb like oregano or garlic, or even citrus fruit, like lemon or lime, which all have a reputation for killing microbes. Also, do not take a probiotic with very hot liquid—for the same reason. If you enjoy a fruit course, take your probiotic with that, since the fermentation of the fruit in the gut facilitates bacterial growth.

Fat

The guidelines from the American Heart Association and the Surgeon General's Office recommend that fat should contribute no more than 30 percent of total calories. Your diet should include more polyunsaturated fat from foods like fish and walnuts, than from the high-cholesterol-producing saturated fat contained in butter, meat, and whole milk. For example, here is the **Polyunsaturated Fat** to **Saturated Fat Ratio** of the breakfast we compared earlier. We try for a 2-to-1 ratio or higher.

CALORIE-RESTRICTED BREAKFAST

Polyunsaturated Fat	Saturated Fat	Ratio
9.03 gm	4.07 gm	2.2 : 1

TYPICAL WESTERN BREAKFAST

Polyunsaturated Fat	Saturated Fat	Ratio
2.77 gm	9.19 gm	0.3 : 1

SET HIGH STANDARDS

To avoid some cardiovascular risk factors, the American Heart Association has set standards that include (1) total blood cholesterol to less than 200 mg/dl, (2) LDL cholesterol in the blood to below 100 mg/dl, (3) HDL cholesterol at a minimum of between 40 and

50 mg/dl for men and between 50 and 60 mg/dl for women, and 4) triglycerides of less than 15 mg/dl. "Healthy" standards for these levels are often based on the idea that if you are within these ranges you are not at risk. But *The CR Way* offers a different perspective. We want more than just perfunctory protection. We want optimal function now and for a long time to come. Therefore, CR practitioners tend to keep their total cholesterol readings in the 150 mg to 160 mg/dl range (or lower), with LDL cholesterol on the low side of 90 mg and HDL cholesterol around 60 mg.

PARAMETER	CALORIE RESTRICTORS	CONTROL GROUP	AHA STANDARDS
Total Cholesterol	158	205	Less than 200
LDL-Cholesterol	91	122	Less than 100 optimal
HDL-Cholesterol	64	50	Men: At least 40 Women: At least 50
Triglycerides	48	147	Less than 150

Data from Washington University studies (Fontana, 2004) compare cardiovascular risk factors of calorie restrictors and a control group, eating a traditional Western diet—shown here alongside the American Heart Association standards (AmericanHeart.org, 2007).

Calorie restrictors who do not achieve great cardiovascular health may be making the wrong food choices. This can be avoided by what you can learn from a medical lab test called Vertical Auto Profile (VAP).

Measures of LDL, HDL, cholesterol, and triglycerides are just rough guides of how healthy a person's heart is. You can ask your doctor for a VAP test that can identify risks that would not be picked up by a normal cholesterol screening. Like the usual cholesterol profile, the VAP test measures total cholesterol, HDL, LDL, and

triglycerides. Where the VAP differs is that it also measures cholesterol subclasses that play important roles in the development of heart
disease. This additional information allows your doctor to improve
the detection of heart disease risk from about 40 percent to 90 percent.

What we especially like about the VAP is that it is sensitive
enough to pick up even small changes in a *CR Way* diet, thus allowing you to tailor your food choices to maximize heart health.

KEEP TRACK

We always recommend keeping track of your food intake so you
can get a sense of how various foods affect you. Simply standing on
the bathroom scale to watch your weight is not enough, especially
when working toward greater cardiovascular health. After you have
measured your food for a while and let your software calculate the
amount of fiber, fats, and the total calorie intake, you will be able to
estimate food amounts when you eat out without having to measure
them on the spot and you will have a good idea what the effects of
that food will be, too.

Although we've tracked our food for years and can accurately
estimate the effects a meal will have, we still keep scales that measure in grams and ounces both in our kitchen and at work. Once we
weigh the food, we enter our intake into our nutrition and fitness
software, NutriBase, which provides many tracking capabilities (see
NutriBase.com); other excellent tracking resources are also available. Try www.calorierestriction.org and NutritionData.com.

LOVING

We can't devote a chapter to the heart without at least a mention of
love. Imagine how romantic it would be if you could take the maturity that time gives you and combine it with a young body that can

respond in lovemaking in much the same way you did when you were in your twenties. Practicing *The CR Way* over the long term makes that possible.

One reason that CR practitioners can retain their ability to express themselves sexually as they get older is that CR increases the body's production of nitric oxide—of principal importance for both male erection and female orgasm. Popular erectile-dysfunction drugs enhance the presence of nitric oxide. But CR folks get it naturally. When you combine the increased nitric oxide production, healthy circulation, optimism, and the energetic way you feel on *The CR Way,* treating a special partner in a more loving way is just natural and your sexual activity will very likely reflect that.

Our recommendation, if you are in a primary relationship, is to talk with your partner about enhancing every aspect of your relationship by travelling *The CR Way* together. You will want to treat each other better. If you are older, you'll find that your ability to express yourselves sexually will become like that of a young couple. You will like what you see when you look in the mirror, too. Those of you who are seniors will begin to see that you both look much younger than your years. And you who can't see the effects of aging yet will postpone those changes. Sharing this with your love partner is a great joy. If you are single and older, on *The CR Way* you will likely feel more confident about becoming intimately involved with someone because you won't have to worry about asking a new partner to understand that your ability to express yourself sexually is—well, not the same as it used to be. Your ability will be abundantly clear.

7

CANCER PREVENTION

Every second about 25 million cells in your body divide. All it takes is one mutation that replicates uncontrolled and then, possibly years later, you discover the frightening effects—a shadow on your lung X-ray, a lump in your breast—and we all know only too well the horrors that follow.

Our environment is full of toxic dangers that can waylay our cells' reproduction mechanisms, shifting them into the overdrive of unbridled cell replication known as cancer. According to the American Cancer Society, a staggering 80 percent of cancers are caused by what's in our environment. But it's not just external forces at work. Our own innate biological systems produce dangerous oxygen molecules known as free radicals that also can cause biological damage that leads to cancer.

You *can* affect this cell reproduction process by paying attention to calorie intake, protein in your diet, the quality of your sleep, carcinogen exposure, exercise, and your stress level. You can help protect yourself against cancer by following *The CR Way*.

The hormesis created by reducing calories shifts the cell

division process into slow motion. Maintaining cell replication at a normal rate doesn't make sense if the body is getting substantially less fuel (calories) than it is used to. The result: Your ability to protect against cancer increases; mutations that lead to cancer are likely to reduce; your body has more time to repair damaged cells and more rapidly kills cells that should be eliminated. In essence, CR greatly reduces the number of cells that are candidates to become cancer.

THE CR WAY TO CANCER PROTECTION

INCREASED CELL PROLIFERATION → SHORTER LIFE

CR WAY
Calorie Restriction decreases IGF-I
Cell division slows

TYPICAL CELL DIVISION
High-calorie or protein intake increases IGF-I
Cell division speeds up

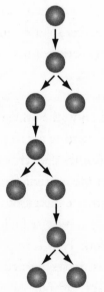
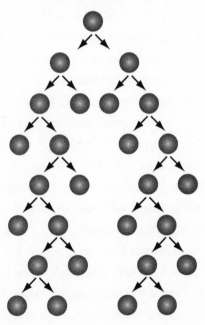

Reduce Rate of Cell Growth

As we saw in Chapter 1, the growth stimulator IGF-I (along with growth hormone and several related molecules) is linked to aging. Laboratory studies consistently show that IGF-I boosts the growth of a variety of cancers, including bladder, breast, lung, colon, stomach, esophageal, liver, pancreatic, kidney, thyroid, brain, ovarian, cervical, and endometrial cancer.

The IGF–cancer link is so strong that some researchers have suggested that IGF-I should be tested along with the standard PSA blood test as a further indicator of prostate cancer risk.

Following a CR plan with moderate protein intake keeps IGF-I and related growth-chemistry low.

Weight Loss and the Immune System

Anyone who wants to prevent cancer and other diseases that involve the immune system needs to understand that dieting brings about immune system changes. It starts with understanding the central role white blood cells play in our body's defenses.

You may remember from high school biology that whenever a germ enters the body the white blood cells go to work to kill it. Some white blood cells produce protective antibodies that overpower the germs, others surround and devour the bacteria. Certain white blood cells specifically attack and destroy cancer cells. Red blood cells help them out.

Maintaining a proper balance of white blood cells is important to your health: High white blood cell levels are associated with leukemia, atherosclerosis, and other diseases, while low white blood cell levels are often associated with anemia. However, a low white blood cell count can also be a sign of fewer immune system challenges (such as inflammation), brought about by CR.

> ## White Blood Cell Count
> (measured in milligrams per deciliter)
>
> Normal range: 4–11.5   CR range: 3–4.5

Several studies have confirmed that dieting often causes the white blood cell count to drop. That's why when a person loses weight, the immune system needs time to adjust. Think of it as an elevator starting on the top floor of a building and your white blood cells are the elevator's passengers. As you lose weight, the elevator descends in slow motion from floor to floor. If you lose weight slowly, the elevator stops at each floor—giving plenty of time for some of your white blood cell passengers to get off. Waiting to get on at each floor are monsters—bacteria, mutant cells, viruses—that want to rush in. As long as the elevator goes slowly, your white blood cells can get off with plenty of time to crowd out all the monsters so none can get on.

But if you decide to lose weight fast, your body cannot adjust quickly enough—meaning that your white blood cell elevator will plunge downward too fast, knocking your protective passengers to the floor. And when the door opens, the monsters will rush in and the white blood cell passengers will engage in a fight to the finish. They may be overwhelmed, because of self-induced overzealous weight loss.

The Right Way to Diet: Slowly

No question: If you are overweight, dropping some pounds is overall a good idea for cancer prevention. In fact, the statistics are overwhelming. So, if you decide to do CR, make sure you start by asking your doctor to order a complete blood count so you know where you stand on important markers like white and red blood cells. See Chapter 8 for lists of what to test. Make sure your doctor explains your results. See Chapter 8 for strategies.

If weight loss is a goal for you on CR or any diet, go slowly—no more than a pound or two a month. Take special care to include in your diet the cancer-prevention foods listed in this chapter as immune system protection along the way.

Cancer's Need for Glucose

In 1931, a Nobel Prize was awarded for the discovery that cancer cells have a fundamentally different energy metabolism from normal cells. Cancer cells were found to need much more glucose than normal cells. Many studies point to high glucose levels as a cancer risk. One study of 1.3 million Koreans found that diabetes and elevated fasting glucose levels were independent risk factors for several major cancers.

The CR Way keeps glucose levels low, a good way to fight the growth of an existing cancer. The case for keeping glucose low to treat cancer is so strong that several biotechnology companies are developing pharmaceuticals that essentially starve cancer cells of glucose.

Many normal cell types have sophisticated energy-producing mechanisms to keep them going when glucose is low. Cancer cells do not. The activation of ketones, as seen in Chapter 5, which is triggered when glucose levels drop, can power normal cells but are essentially unusable for cancer cells. Starved of the glucose energy they need, cancer cells cannot easily proliferate.

Insulin: Also a Risk

Throughout this book when we talk about glucose control in healthy people, we are also talking about insulin control. While glucose provides the energy a tumor needs, insulin activates growth factors that make it possible for the tumor to grow and replicate.

Insulin, you'll remember, is a balance to glucose: When too much glucose is available, insulin levels surge to process it. And we've seen that high glucose, and the accompanying insulin, can accelerate aging. While measuring insulin levels requires a trip to the laboratory, glucose is easily measured by anyone willing to use a blood glucose meter. Therefore, for practical everyday management of insulin levels, measuring glucose is the way to go. While glucose provides the energy a tumor needs to grow, insulin activates the growth factors that make it possible for the tumor to grow and replicate.

Numerous studies have linked high insulin levels to cancer incidence and to poorer outcomes once cancer is diagnosed. One very impressive ten-year study followed 535 women with newly diagnosed breast cancer. While some in the study were obese, others were of normal weight or slim. Regardless of these weight differences, higher insulin levels corresponded to reduced survival rates.

The women who had the best survival and recurrence outcomes had low fasting insulin levels, which ranged from 2.0 microIU/ml to 3.3 microIU/ml. Fasting levels of insulin in CR practitioners are often even lower than these (about 1.6 in the Wash. U. cohort). Although this breast cancer study did not focus on CR, the low insulin levels achieved on *The CR Way* clearly match the findings that low insulin levels helped protect participants against cancer recurrence.

Keep Abdominal Fat Low

As we get older, the fat distribution in our bodies changes, and for many people that means fat accumulation in the abdominal area. A high percentage of body fat is already a risk factor for diabetes, cancer, and heart disease, but abdominal fat adds insult to injury.

Your chances of getting cancer and other major diseases soar and your chances of surviving a disease plunge.

CR protects against fat accumulation by burning fat for energy. CR by itself has produced impressive declines in overall body fat that will help protect against abdominal fat accumulation.

People with a high waist-to-hip ratio, where the waist measure is equal to or larger than the hip, typically have an apple shape, with fat concentrated in the abdomen. One study of risk for invasive breast cancer found that women with a waist-to-hip ratio greater than 0.80, indicating higher concentrations of abdominal fat, were 52 percent more likely to die of breast cancer in the next nine years compared to those with ratios at or below 0.80, after adjusting for the effects of obesity.

The study also showed that obesity has a detrimental effect on breast cancer survival. Women with a Body Mass Index greater than 30, which indicates obesity, were 48 percent more likely to die during the nine-year study period than women of ideal weight. When the study participants were both overweight (Body Mass Index greater than 25) and had a waist-to-hip ratio above 0.80, their risk of dying increased by 92 percent.

IS YOUR BODY FAT A RISK?

According to the U.S. Department of Health and Human Services, excess body fat leads to higher risk for premature death and disease including Type II diabetes, high blood pressure, cardiovascular disease, and cancer. The Body Mass Index (BMI), based on height and weight, is often used to approximate body fat.

Use the following chart as an approximate guide to body fat status. However, take into account that BMI overestimates body fat in people with high muscle mass and underestimates it in people who have lost muscle mass.

Some foods, when consumed in excess, can cause extra waist fat:

- Carbohydrate from refined grains and potatoes
- Foods containing simple sugars
- Vegetable fat
- Alcohol

(Halkjaer, 2005)

A diet emphasizing fruits and vegetables like the complex carbs recommended on *The CR Way* may help to reduce waist size.

ADULT BMI CHART

BMI	19	20	21	22	23	24	25	26	27	28	29	30	31	32	33	34	35
Height	**Weight in Pounds**																
4'10"	91	96	100	105	110	115	119	124	129	134	138	143	148	153	158	162	167
4'11"	94	99	104	109	114	119	124	128	133	138	143	148	153	158	163	168	173
5'	97	102	107	112	118	123	128	133	138	143	148	153	158	163	168	174	179
5'1"	100	106	111	116	122	127	132	137	143	148	153	158	164	169	174	180	185
5'2"	104	409	115	120	126	131	136	142	147	153	158	164	169	175	180	186	191
5'3"	107	113	118	124	130	135	141	146	152	158	163	169	175	180	186	191	197
5'4"	110	116	122	128	134	140	145	151	157	163	169	174	180	186	192	197	204
5'5"	114	120	123	132	138	144	150	156	162	168	174	180	186	192	198	204	210
5'6"	118	124	130	136	142	148	155	161	167	173	179	186	192	198	204	210	216
5'7"	121	127	134	140	146	153	159	166	172	178	185	191	198	204	211	217	223
5'8"	125	131	138	144	151	158	164	171	177	184	190	197	203	210	216	223	230
5'9"	128	135	142	149	155	162	169	176	182	189	196	203	209	216	223	230	236
5'10"	132	139	146	153	160	167	174	181	188	195	202	209	216	222	229	236	243
5'11"	136	143	150	157	165	172	179	186	193	200	208	215	222	229	236	243	250
6'	140	147	154	162	169	177	184	191	199	206	213	221	228	235	242	250	258
6'1"	144	151	159	166	174	182	189	197	204	212	219	227	235	242	250	257	265
6'2"	148	155	163	171	179	186	194	202	210	218	225	233	241	249	256	264	272
6'3"	152	160	168	176	184	192	200	208	216	224	232	240	248	256	264	272	279
	Healthy Weight						**Overweight**					**Obese**					

U.S. Department of Health and Human Services
Dietary Guidelines for Americans, 2005

Avoid Carcinogens

With 80 percent of cancers estimated to be caused by environmental exposure, part of your anticancer strategy must be to avoid as many carcinogens as possible.

The CR Way is about optimal living. While we are all exposed to carcinogens in our environment, we have more control over what we take into our bodies—we can minimize the hazards by watching what we eat.

Organic

Nonorganic pesticides, extra hormones, and other substances that may cause cancer or wreak havoc on our immune systems are often contained in commercially prepared foods and used in conventional methods of growing fruits and vegetables. So why take the risk? On *The CR Way*, we seek out organic foods and limit food intake that is not organic.

Not all organic foods are automatically safe. Some organic produce has a higher rate of bacterial infestation than conventionally grown produce. Look carefully for any sign of mold on produce and reject it immediately if you even have to question it. Many advocates of organic foods offer elaborate cleaning methods for removing bacteria, such as washing produce with salt water or bathing it in mild bleach solutions. Washing produce in caustic chemicals may cause the plant to absorb toxic residue, canceling out the value of buying organic. Besides, the bacteria don't necessarily stay on the outside of fruit and vegetables. They often work their way down the stem of the fruit to its core. They can also be absorbed from the soil that has been contaminated by years of nonorganic agricultural chemical use.

Our simple solution is to cook all foods except frozen berries. According to the Centers for Disease Control, heating food to an internal temperature above 160°F, or 78°C, **for even a few seconds** will kill parasites, viruses, and almost all bacteria. Boiling is the best way to kill most food microbes—from a thirty-second blanch for fruits or nuts to five minutes or more for denser vegetables. Cutting foods into small pieces facilitates the process. Adding lemon or lime juice to food also helps keep the microbial count down.

Cancer-Preventing foods
Functional Food

The crux of *The CR Way* has always been to pack every calorie we eat with the most nutrition we can: no empty calories, only calories full of vitamins, minerals, and/or phytochemicals.

> ## Phytochemicals
>
> Phytochemicals are plant substances that are not vitamins or essential nutrients but are known to have beneficial health effects.

A great example is blueberries. Twelve years ago, they weren't very strong on our radar, since the amounts of vitamins and minerals they contain are rather modest compared to those of some other fruits. Now blueberries are a top pick due to phytochemicals that are associated with promoting better memory. Antioxidants and inflammation reduction are also valuable benefits. Other foods with cancer-fighting qualities include almost all the food choices in the Foods to Choose chapter, including favorites like walnuts, raspberries, barley, and onions.

Blueberries for Longer Life

A study by the National Institute on Aging has found that polyphenols in blueberries increased lifespan and slowed aging-related functional declines. *(Lau, 2005)*

A University of Barcelona study found the flavonoids in blueberries can reverse age-related neural deficits and may enhance memory.
(Andrea-Lacueva, 2005)

Building on the *CR Way* basics of reduced calories, low glucose, and moderate protein intake that we've shown fight cancer—another level of protection is available from the array of delicious, healthful foods to choose.

Color Us Healthy

Like an artist choosing from an array of colors for a painting, you can vary the colors of your foods every day for your cancer-prevention program. The colors of vegetables and fruits reflect their phytochemical content and thus their disease-preventing benefits; for example:

Red:

Lycopene gives tomatoes and red peppers their characteristic red color. Lycopene is linked to preventing prostate, colon, rectal and stomach cancer, and possibly also breast and cervical cancers.

Green:

Sulforaphanes impart a gorgeous green color to vegetables like broccoli and Brussels sprouts, and are linked to mobilizing the liver's detoxification enzymes, which neutralize dangerous cancer-causing chemicals before they can damage DNA and promote cancer.

Blue:

Anthocyanins make blueberries blue. Actually their pigments are responsible for the red, purple, and blue colors of many fruits and vegetables. **Anthocyanins** are powerful antioxidants that may protect against colon and esophageal cancers, and that can increase visual acuity and improve circulatory disorders.

White/Green:

Organosulfides, found in garlic and onions, have been shown to fight a variety of cancers and possibly prevent benzopyrenes, produced by some cooking methods, from having their cancer-causing effect in the body.

Green/Orange:

Zeaxanthin and Lutein—two carotenoids found in many green vegetables, orange peppers, and egg yolks—may help stave off the toxic reaction on healthy cells caused by drugs used in chemotherapy. Both have been linked to prevention of breast and prostate cancers.

FOOD SUGGESTIONS TO *COLOR **YOU** HEALTHY* ON *THE CR WAY*

FRUIT

Yellow	Lemon juice
Red	Strawberries
Blue, red, purple	Blueberries and raspberries

VEGGIES

Yellow	Ginger, yellow peppers
Red	Tomatoes, red peppers, sweet potato
Green	Broccoli, green peppers, spinach, and other greens, like Swiss chard and kale
White-green	Onion, cauliflower, garlic

Some Cancer-Fighting Foods

Mushroom Magic for the Immune System

Maitake and shiitake mushrooms provide valuable immune system benefits and both have been shown to possess anticarcinogenic properties.

Maitake, available by mail order and at some supermarkets, in Japanese means the "dancing mushroom" because people were said to dance for joy when they happened to discover a large maitake mushroom in the wild. Maitake is known to be a powerful immune system stimulant, activating various effector cells that attack tumors.

Shiitake mushrooms are readily available in many groceries and health food stores. They have been shown to have anticancer effects on colon and prostate cancers and on leukemia, as well as to impede cell mutation caused by carcinogens.

On *The CR Way* we combine either of these mushrooms with

onion, leafy vegetables like mustard greens, along with turnips or kohlrabi to make a delicious cancer-prevention soup we enjoy several times a week.

Onions and Garlic: Effective Against Cancer and High Blood Sugar

Onion and garlic are a perfect fit on *The CR Way* by lowering cholesterol, reducing blood pressure and the risk of blood clots. If you are taking a blood thinner, be especially careful about adding large amounts of these vegetables to your diet, given their own blood-thinning potential.

Garlic may also increase the immune system's effectiveness in attacking tumors. Studies suggest that regular garlic and onion intake reduces the risk of developing several types of cancer: Stomach, intestinal, and ovarian cancer were reduced by both garlic and onion in laboratory studies. Prostate, nasopharyngeal, and colorectal cancer cells were reduced by garlic.

Research data showed that the more onion and garlic people ate per week, the less likely they were to be diagnosed with a whole range of cancers. The researchers concluded: Making onion and garlic staples in a healthful way of eating may greatly lower the risk of several common cancers. (Galeone, 2006)

Lemon and Lime

The juices of these two fruits are an important part of *The CR Way*. Unlike most fruit juices, which cause spikes of glucose into the bloodstream, the juices of these fruits actually lower glucose absorption from a meal, making it easier to keep your glucose levels low to help prevent cancer. Either fruit may also help kill unfriendly bacteria. The bioflavonoids contained in the skin of these fruits work with vitamin C to maintain healthy capillaries, heal wounds, and form collagen in connective tissue.

Barley

Barley is high in the indigestible fiber (known as beta-glucan) that may increase the activity of white blood cell components to fight cancer. Inspiration for using beta glucans to treat cancer comes from animal studies showing that beta glucans increase tumor regression.

Barley ranks low on the Glycemic Index, making it another great food for keeping glucose low. Barley has a very beneficial effect on the colon in that the indigestible fiber it contains helps form short-chain fatty acids that have many beneficial health effects including:

- Stabilizing blood glucose levels
- Lowering cholesterol
- Protecting and strengthening the colon lining
- Improving immune function
- Increasing beneficial bacteria in intestine

Include barley in meals several times a week or even every day—combined with vegetables, olive oil, and lemon juice. Warm it in vegetable broth to make a delicious soup that adds a wonderful functional food to your CR diet.

To enrich your diet with more cancer-fighting foods, see the food chart on page 160.

PART III

THE PLAN

8

GETTING STARTED ON *THE CR WAY*

BEFORE YOU BEGIN

The CR Way can be adapted to fit any lifestyle.

The old saying may be "you are what you eat," but in reality you are so much more. To get the most benefit from the program, begin by completing this personal health assessment. Then use the suggestions in the chapter to customize *The CR Way* to your individual needs.

MY PERSONAL PROFILE

Today's date:
Age:
Height (inches):
Weight (pounds):
Waist size (inches):
BMI (Body Mass Index):

Use the BMI chart in Chapter 7 or use this formula:

Weight in pounds ÷ Height in inches × Height in inches × 703.

My BMI indicates that I am:

❑ Underweight
❑ On target with CR averages (18 to 21.4)
❑ Normal weight
❑ Overweight
❑ Obese

Determine Your Disease Risk

Your disease risk depends on your family's history of diseases and your own personal health parameters. This is extremely valuable information, because understanding both your own conditions that may put you in danger and your heritable disease risks allows you to take steps to guard against them. You'll get the details of your health parameters when you meet with your doctor for your physical. And he or she can tell you the significance of your family history, which you should complete and take with you to your doctor visit.

Family History

Are your parents and/or grandparents alive?
If not, what did your parents die from and at what age?

If not, what did your grandparents die from and at what age?
Maternal grandmother:
Maternal grandfather:
Paternal grandmother:
Paternal grandfather:
Do you have any brothers or sisters or children? Are they fit and well?

A family history of some diseases increases your risk for that disease.

> Have you a family history of:
>
> Autoimmune disorders
>
> Neurological decline, e.g., diseases such as Alzheimer's and Parkinson's
>
> Heart attack or stroke
>
> Diabetes
>
> High blood pressure
>
> Cancer
>
> > Type of cancer
>
> Fracture/osteoporosis in your immediate family, including grandparents

What are your personal risk factors?

> High blood pressure (hypertension)
>
> High LDL cholesterol ("bad" cholesterol)
>
> Low HDL cholesterol ("good" cholesterol)
>
> High triglycerides
>
> High body fat
>
> High (above 100) blood glucose (sugar)
>
> Depression
>
> Physical inactivity
>
> Carcinogen exposure
>
> Tobacco smoking

Compiling this information will allow you to focus on your current lifestyle as well as any health factors that might pose a risk. This will prepare you for your doctor visit and help you get the most from it.

Your Relationship with Your Doctor

Establish a good relationship with at least one doctor who (1) understands calorie restriction or is willing to learn with you and (2) is interested enough in working with you to make sure your journey on *The CR Way* is healthy. Your physician should be willing to help you decide what to test, share test results, and explain anything you don't understand.

Your family doctor or internist, or whoever is your primary care physician, is a prime candidate. We also work with an endocrinologist, who takes a personal interest in our research. Make sure you get copies of your lab results, not just a note from the doctor, saying everything is okay.

Once you discuss CR with the doctor, your job is to make it easy for him or her to help you. A topnotch physician, like the one you are going to select, will have many patients. Your second job is to get the doctor to really focus on you. To help channel his or her attention, we recommend that you send a letter to the physician in advance of your appointment, highlighting your intentions and the tests you would like to have done.

Sample Physician Letter

Dear Doctor:

I have decided to pursue the most scientifically researched way to avoid disease and increase my chances to live longer: calorie restriction with optimal nutrition.

My plan is to lose [fill in . . . (only if you plan to lose weight)] pounds over the next [fill in time period]. Upon achieving my weight goal, I will increase my calories enough to maintain my BMI at my new, healthy level.

[*Note: If your physician is unfamiliar with the science and the health benefits of calorie restriction, you may direct him or her to several scientific papers, including:*

Fontana L. "Excessive adiposity, calorie restriction, and aging." *JAMA.* **2006** Apr 5; 295(13):1577–8. PMID: 16595760.

Fontana L, Meyer TE, Klein S, Holloszy JO. "Long-term calorie restriction is highly effective in reducing the risk for atherosclerosis in humans." *Proceedings of the National Academy of Sciences* **2004** Apr 27; 101(17):6659–63. PMID: 15096581.]

Before I start, I need to thoroughly assess my health status so I can accurately gauge my progress. Please let your office staff know that I will be calling to schedule a complete physical, along with the following blood work:

[Include here the CR Benchmarks Panel on pages 146–47.]

Please be so kind as to share the actual results of those tests with me—including the lab printouts so I can enter them into the spreadsheet that I will be using to track my progress.

I would like to make sure I test the same indicators again after six months into my program to gauge my progress.

[*If you take medication or have health conditions, include the following:*]

As you know, I am taking the following medications and am currently being treated for:

Would any of these medications or conditions be adversely affected by caloric restriction?

Thank you,

NEXT STEPS ON *THE CR WAY*

Step One

Know what to eat

Limiting calories doesn't mean you must limit taste or variety in your foods. Common sense will often dictate the kinds of healthy, highly nutritious selections you'll make—vitamin-rich vegetables, nutrient-packed grains and legumes, beans, berries, and a host of herbs and spices are all among your bountiful choices.

We've provided an extensive list of Foods to Choose in the next chapter and encourage you to experiment with flavors and textures when preparing your meals. Use our recipes and meal suggestions to guide you and you'll discover you are limited only by your imagination.

Journey on *The CR Way*

Imagine taking a journey to a new place without directions. Would you arrive at the right destination?

Your journey on *The CR Way* comes with easy-to-follow directions to guide you toward a long, healthy life.

The two most important:

1. Visit your doctor before beginning and have your medical testing done (see the CR Benchmarks section in this chapter).
2. Track your food intake to stay on course.

Step Two

Know how many calories you are eating

To know how many calories you are taking in, you need to weigh your food. This may sound like a lot of work at first, but it is really not nearly as time-consuming as you might think. Once you get the hang of weighing, you'll find that you do it automatically and it doesn't really slow you down.

Use a digital scale to weigh food in grams or ounces. We keep a scale in our kitchen that measures in both and converts to the other at the touch of a button. This makes tracking easy because food labels can be in either unit. Thinking in grams may seem strange at first, but once you get used to it, dietary tracking will be much easier because the databases—like the big one from the USDA, http://www.nal.usda.gov/fnic/foodcomp/search—usually use grams. Kitchen scales are available in some stores and on the Internet. We prefer stainless steel scales with removable platform covers that are easy to clean. Moderately priced models are available with a reading range of 1 gram (0.1 ounce) to 7 kilograms (15.4 pounds) capacity. Some measure in grams and ounces, ounces and pounds; pounds and kilograms—anything you need for measuring food.

Step Three

Track your food intake

Once you weigh what you eat, you are halfway to making a major difference in your health. The next step is to enter your intake into a diary or preferably good dietary-tracking software that will calculate your total calorie intake and give you a detailed breakdown of everything your diet supplies, so you know what you are really getting. Dr. Walford's Interactive Diet Planner (DWIDP) is a free download for members of the Calorie Restriction Society (www.calorierestriction.org); NutriBase offers software at several levels of capability and cost. At www.NutriBase.com, you can also learn about NutriBase's competition.

NutriBase is updated frequently with the latest USDA Nutrient Database for Standard Reference, along with the Canadian Nutrient Files, and many entries for manufactured products.

You won't have to waste time looking up a food every time you want to enter it either. Software programs allow development of a list of favorite foods that makes it easy to enter your choices even when you are in a hurry. In fact, if we know we are going to include certain items in our meals every day, we can enter them into the auto-record feature and they automatically appear on the intake screen—reducing the bother of reentering them every day.

If you decide to keep a paper diary, it should look something like this:

Date:					
Food item	Food item weight	Total calories	Carbohy-drate calories	Fat calories	Protein calories
Totals/meal (at the end of each meal's entries)					
Totals/day (at the end of the day's entries)					
Totals/day					

Where the Entries Come From

You know the food item. The labels of most nonproduce foods list the calories per serving, often even the calories from the three macronutrients: carbohydrates, fat, and protein. You weigh a serving for yourself and record it, along with the calorie listings—and you're done. If you want more or less than the serving size listed, we recommend that you alter the amount in fractions of the serving size, so you can take advantage of the caloric analysis that's already been done by the manufacturer.

Tracking Made Easy

In our kitchen, we keep a laptop computer for the purpose of tracking our food intake. That way, entering our intake is almost as easy as getting something out of the refrigerator.

When you are recording produce, the nutrition data are available online at the USDA Web site http://www.nal.usda.gov/fnic/food-comp/search.

In addition to tracking nutrients, tracking your caloric expenditure from exercise is also valuable, as well as tracking glucose, cholesterol, blood pressure, and a host of other markers that will enable you to see changes and trends.

When we first started recording our food intake, it was a real eye-opener. We thought our diet was the best it could be, but we were missing several important nutrients and eating more calories than we thought. If you are not using a computer, keeping your food intake in a diary will definitely help, but you will have to do some fancy arithmetic to make all the calculations that this software does instantly. The analyses in Chapters 4 (page 72) and 6 (pages 102, and 104), as well as the following provide examples of what our software program can do. It gives us instant, in-depth readouts of what our diet really provides. Here is an example of a complete analysis of the model meal in Chapter 4.

Morning Tease Meal, 88 Calories

	CONVENTIONAL MEASURES	GRAMS	CALORIES
Sweet potato	¼ cup	70	53
Olive oil	1 teaspoon	4	36

Breakfast Main Meal, 805 Calories (For recipes, see Chapter 10)

	CONVENTIONAL MEASURES	GRAMS	CALORIES
Lemon-Ginger Salmon	3½ ounces	100	147
Potluck Vegetable Soup			
(weight of vegetables)	1 cup (scant)	200	84
Savory Barley *(enjoyably combined with salmon and/or soup)*	1½ cups	375	324
The CR Way Dressing	3 tablespoons	21	84
Lentils and tomatoes	½ cup	120	102
Raspberries and	½ cup	120	51
walnuts	3 halves	6	39

TOTAL NUTRIENT INTAKE: MODEL MEAL (INCLUDING TEASE AND MAIN MEAL)

Total calories	893
Carbohydrate-Protein-Fat ratio	59-14-27
Protein (gm)	33
Total lipid (fat) (gm)	28
Fatty acids, saturated (gm)	4
Fatty acids, monounsaturated (gm)	15
Fatty acids, polyunsaturated (gm)	6
Omega-3 (gm)	1.9
Omega-6 (gm)	3.7
Cholesterol (mg)	60

Phytosterols (mg)	43
Sugars, total (gm)	28
Glucose (gm)	1.5
Fructose (gm)	1
Fiber, total dietary (gm)	32

VITAMINS

Vitamin A (IU)	13,117
Vitamin B-1, Thiamin (mg)	3.77
Vitamin B-2, Riboflavin (mg)	3.7
Vitamin B-3, Niacin (mg)	10
Vitamin B-5, Pantothenic acid (mg)	2
Vitamin B-6 (mg)	1.1
Total Folate (mcg)	164
Vitamin B-12, Cobalamin (mcg)	3.1
Vitamin C, Ascorbic acid (mg)	91.7
Alpha-tocopherol (IU)	3
Gamma-tocopherol (IU)	1.2
Vitamin E (IU)	2.9

MINERALS

Calcium, Ca (mg)	363
Copper, Cu (mg)	.68
Iron, Fe (mg)	8.8
Magnesium, Mg (mg)	136
Manganese, Mn (mg)	1.6
Phosphorus, P (mg)	619
Potassium, K (mg)	1488
Selenium, Se (mcg)	42
Sodium, Na (mg)	216
Zinc, Zn (mg)(supplement)	3.5

This model meal probably seems like a lot of food. And it is! But remember, the *total* calories you eat during the day determine whether you are calorie restricted or not. And this is the bigger of our two meals. We eat this higher-calorie meal in the morning and a smaller yet substantial lunch filled with taste treats like those found in the recipes in this book—lemon-ginger sweet potatoes, an open-faced sandwich of green bean spread and veggies on spouted-grain bread, or a barley-and-vegetable soup, for example. We then enjoy fasting for the rest of the day. Paul's total calories will be around 1900 and Meredith's around 1600—all jam-packed with nutrients. By the end of the day the totals will supply 100 percent or more of the DRI of vitamins, minerals, and amino acids—plus many valuable phytochemicals.

What If You Don't Want to Track?

Because *The CR Way* is truly for everybody and anybody, you should do what feels most comfortable. We happen to be very interested in knowing the effects of everything we eat, so tracking fits our style of calorie restriction perfectly. But some of the world's most successful calorie restrictors do not measure their food. The ones we know, however, watch their weight carefully and visit their doctors regularly. The key to their success is that as they get older and their bodies slow down, they are careful to cut their food intake so they do not gain weight.

Ralph, our friend and CR mentor, lived for 104 productive and joyful years and practiced CR *very successfully* for his last 50 years. He never tracked his intake except with morning weighing and trips to his doctor. When an interviewer asked about exercise, his response was, "Oh, yes—the thumb exercise is the most important. That's the one where you push yourself away from the table when you *start* to get full."

Become an Expert on How Food Affects You

Just like an expert jeweler who can distinguish between fake and real gold, by tracking the food you eat, you will become an expert on how food affects you—good or bad. Do you know how a meal of your favorite carbohydrate foods affects your blood sugar? How does salt intake affect your blood pressure? Answers to questions like these will become second nature. Estimating how many calories various foods are really giving you will also become easy and particularly helpful when you are eating out.

Step Four

Measuring Your Success

To whatever degree you choose to follow *The CR Way*, doing some tracking will help you enormously. The truth is, if you don't track any of the changes you are making and their effects, you won't know which foods, supplements, exercises, meditation practices, and so forth really work for you. So here are some of the most useful measures to track:

* Measure glucose

In Chapter 4, we saw the importance of measuring glucose—to provide a quick and easy assessment of not only circulating glucose, but also probable insulin levels, and maybe even SIRT1 expression—three pillars of successful CR.

To measure glucose, select a glucose meter that's pain-free: www.Mendosa.com provides an in-depth comparison of the meters on the market.

Measuring with a glucose meter is also the key to living the low-glucose lifestyle that leads to increased energy (Chapter 1), protection against AGE (Chapter 4), and increased cognitive abilities (Chapter 5).

* Measure body temperature, blood pressure, and heart rate

Body Temperature May Predict Longevity

In a study by the NIA, perceptive researchers looked at male participants in the Baltimore Longitudinal Study of Aging (BLSA), which began in 1958.

Three markers that have been shown to predict lifespan in laboratory animals turned out to be predictors of BLSA subject longevity: lower body temperature, lower circulating insulin, and higher levels of the hormone DHEAS.

Roth, 2002

Body temperature is lowered by CR. This is easy to measure at home and something we often track. Make sure you measure at the same time of day and under the same indoor conditions to reduce the variables that affect your readings. To calculate what your average is, be sure to take readings on several days before you start CR. This gives you a baseline to track the effects of *The CR Way*.

And always take your temperature orally or always take it rectally. Oral and rectal thermometers are easy to get at drugstores. For most healthy individuals, the average body temperature is 98.2 degrees Fahrenheit. Our own body temperatures average between 96.5° F and 97° F, typical for calorie restrictors. Your average body temperature's decrease with CR may indicate a slower metabolic rate, which scientists speculate results in fewer cell-attacking free radicals and ultimately less genetic damage.

Having a blood pressure monitor at home is also a great idea. As you implement even small changes in your diet, you will likely be delighted that your heart rate and blood pressure also begin to fall. Just adding fish oil alone will likely produce a measurable blood pressure drop. Tracking blood pressure at the same time you are recording dietary intake is also a good way to see how your blood pressure responds to salt intake.

*Measure body fat

One of the most amazing aspects of the first few years on CR was watching our body fat melt away. Because body fat is such a strong predictor of disease and overall indicator of inflammation status, it is definitely important to track. Our bathroom scale automatically provides an estimate of body fat. Many products are available for this purpose, including calipers, tape measures, hand-held devices, and various types of bathroom scales.

Step Five

Measure strength, endurance, and smarts

Have you ever watched a pitcher at a ball game who is having a great day? Everything goes right. His fastball blazes across the plate and batter after batter strikes out. Professional athletes definitely know when they are "on" because of the athletic challenges they give their bodies.

Knowing how "on" you are is extremely useful. You can learn this by doing physical and mental exercises regularly.

Physical Fitness

Physical exercise is an important, healthful component of *The CR Way*, but like everything we do, moderation is the key. Our culture puts a premium on instant gratification, and when it comes to our bodies, we want to see fast results. However, the combination of restricting calories and overexerting with intense exercise can put undue stress on your immune system, possibly creating serious danger. Intense exercise depresses the immune system in humans, and it increases inflammation—exactly the opposite of the effect CR gives us.

Moderate Exercise Routines

Take a 30–50-minute walk every day. We take one in place of eating dinner and find it's a great time to share conversation and enjoy the scenery or sunset.

Lift weights. Exercising each muscle group with the heaviest weight you can lift—two sets and a maximum of 12 repetitions per set, twice weekly—will help maintain joint strength and possibly protect against osteoporosis.

Yoga. The stretching and breathing are excellent ways to start or end your day, and you'll strengthen your core muscles, too.

Walking with weights. A weight belt or vest will make you work a little harder as you walk, tricking your body into thinking it is heavier. This will help stop age-related loss of bone density.

Rest. Listen to your body and don't overdo it. No matter how much exercise you planned, if you feel exceptionally tired or your performance is slightly under par—cut it short that day and give yourself some extra rest.

The good news, however, is that moderate exercise can increase the production of the white blood cells that attack bacteria, and regular moderate exercise can substantially benefit the immune system over the long term.

Strength building: Building strong muscles and bones through weight-lifting exercises twice a week, as well as exercising regularly with a weight vest will help protect against osteoporosis. A particularly exciting study (Snow, 2000) has shown that older postmenopausal women who wore weighted vests and engaged in jumping exercises three times per week for thirty-two weeks of the year over a five-year period did not lose significant bone density. This is directly relevant to slim people, who are at greater risk of osteoporosis: The less weight the bones are challenged to carry, the less density they maintain.

Exercise as an effectiveness gauge: Adjust your exercise program to fit your new life. You can also use your exercise routine as a gauge of the effectiveness of your *CR Way* lifestyle. If you perform below your peak on only one day, think nothing of it and just do fewer repetitions. If you perform below your peak on several days and/ or decline steadily, that should be a warning signal. Consider whether you are trying to lift too heavy a weight too soon or not giving your muscles enough rest between workouts—exercising each muscle group twice a week is optimal. Also look carefully at your daily food intake to ensure that you are not limiting calories or protein too much, and make sure you are getting enough sleep.

Aerobic exercise: Regular, moderate aerobic exercise is an important element of any lifestyle, and this is true of *The CR Way*. Great for heart health, it can also be an effective way to help reduce stress. We run, row, and do a few other moderate aerobic exercises regularly. Again, think nothing of it if you suddenly huff and puff one day while engaging in your usual routine. Just make sure to adjust. Don't push it—relax and cut the session short. But if you cannot sustain your normal level of exercise or become winded quickly, see a doctor right away just to double-check to make sure your heart is okay.

Brain Fitness

Like physical exercise, your brain can and should be exercised to increase cognitive abilities. Learning a foreign language has gained a deserved reputation for being good for brain fitness. Learning to play a musical instrument and probably anything else that requires learning new skills will benefit your cognitive health. Especially when you use a skills test that challenges you to perform at your peak, you will know right away if you are up to par. *The CR Way* includes mental exercises that allow for quantifiable results—computer packages of mental proficiency tests, for example.

The point of all of these exercises is to put you in touch with your body in a most sensitive way. As you record your foods, sleep well, and do all the healthful things that make up *The CR Way*, you will become acutely sensitive to what affects you and helps you live your life fully.

Step Six

Focus on Good Health and Longevity, not Weight Loss

Although measuring calories and tracking weight is what may come to mind first when people think of CR, no one really knows what *the* ideal weight is. Nor does anyone know the ideal number of calories a person should take in to be optimally calorie restricted—in part because these are different for each individual.

Calorie restriction is intended as a way to extend our lives in the healthiest way possible, not a quick fix for dropping a few pounds. By identifying your personal goals and tracking your calories, glucose, and protein, you will learn about your own optimal food intake and balance it with exercise, meditation, and other healthful lifestyle choices. Still, although CR is not a weight-loss plan, calorie restrictors usually lose weight. Losing more weight than you want to is all too easy if you are already at a healthy weight.

The most fundamental thing to understand about CR is what is actually going on inside your cells—the beneficial impact that hormesis has on slowing your body's aging process. The number on your bathroom scale is incidental to the biological markers, which can be tested at your local lab, in telling you how healthy you are. The chances are that if these biomarkers found in your blood test results are already close to the CR averages we list in this section, you don't need to lose weight and your dietary choices are already close to what you need.

However, if your averages are not close to these numbers, start by changing your dietary selections, using the Foods to Choose chapter. Just by changing your food choices you will probably begin to lose some weight, since it is easy to fill up on low-calorie food. And more to the point, your biomarkers will begin to change.

Next, set goals that will put your weight, body fat, and circulating glucose (Chapter 4) somewhere near the averages in *The CR Way* Benchmarks Panel on pages 146–47. And for the sake of your immune system (see Chapter 7), if your weight is far from the average listed, lose weight slowly over a period of a year or more, not months. Do the same with circulating glucose. There is no need to go from dangerously high levels to the 80s or below at breakneck speed. Do it over a period of a month or more.

Once you achieve your weight and body fat goals, make that your **line-in-the-sand** level. Don't ever go below it unless you have a very good health-related and doctor-approved reason. If you cross your line-in-the-sand number, do not rationalize it and reset your weight and fat goals lower and lower. Stop restricting calories and gradually eat more of the good, nutrient-dense food that you love until you get back above your line.

The CR Way Benchmarks Panel

How can you know if the hormesis of CR is really working in your body?

Let *The CR Way* Benchmarks Panel be your guide. These tests should be included in the complete physical you get when you start CR. Your results will give you a baseline to judge future progress. As you proceed on CR, you can periodically use *The CR Way* Benchmarks Panel to gauge just how well your plan is working.

THE CR WAY BENCHMARKS PANEL

CARDIOVASCULAR
Lipids
> Total cholesterol, mg/dl
> LDL-C, mg/dl
> HDL-C, mg/dl
> Triglycerides, mg/dl

> Instead of the standard lipid profile, do consider using the VAP—Vertical Auto Profile—complete lipid profile, including subparticles that are risk factors (see Chapter 6).

Blood pressure
> Systolic BP, mmHg
> Diastolic BP, mmHg

Heart status
> Electrocardiogram (detects heart problems or blockages in the coronary arteries and measures heartbeat regularity and rate)
> Echocardiogram (tests status of heart muscle)

IMMUNE STATUS
> hsCRP, mg/L, one of the best predictors of heart attack
> TNF-alpha, pg/ml

GLUCOSE AND INSULIN
Fasting glucose, mg/dl
Fasting insulin, microIU/ml

COMPLETE BLOOD COUNT
Provides important information about the kinds and numbers of
cells in the blood, especially
Red blood cells (RBC)
White blood cells (WBC)
Platelets

METABOLIC PANEL
Calcium   Protein   Electrolytes
Kidney status   Liver status

OSTEOPOROSIS RISK
DEXA (measures bone density status)

THYROID HORMONES
T3 regulates most thyroid actions (ng/dl)

GROWTH STATUS
IGF-I–Insulin-like Growth Factor-I (ng/ml)

Following is a log where you can track your scores alongside
actual results compiled from human CR studies at Washington
University School of Medicine in Saint Louis. If you aim for these
numbers, you'll almost certainly be on the right track.

THE CR WAY BENCHMARKS PANEL
PERSONAL LOG

	CR GROUP WASH. U.	YOUR SCORES NOW	YOUR SCORES IN 6 MONTHS	YOUR SCORES IN 1 YEAR
Age (yrs)	40–64			
Sex (M/F)	24 Male 4 Female			
Height (feet and inches)	5' 4"–6'0"			
Weight (pounds)	114.4–140.8			
BMI (weight: height)*	18.5–21.4			
Total cholesterol, mg/dl	119–197			
LDL-C, mg/dl	58–114			
HDL-C, mg/dl	44–82			
Triglycerides, mg/dl	33–63			
Systolic BP, mmHg	89–109			
Diastolic BP, mmHg	55–67			
Fasting glucose, mg/dl	74–88			
Fasting insulin, mIU/ml	0.6–2.2			
T3 (ng/dl)	51.6–95.6			
hsCRP (mg/L)	0.1–0.5			
TNF-alpha (pg/ml)	0.24–1.24			
HRest (beats/min)	48–64			
IGF-I (ng/mL)	102–178			

*Although some in the CR group tested a bit lower, it is not recommended.

Congratulations for getting started on *The CR Way!*
See you at your *100th birthday* party.

9

FOODS TO CHOOSE

Imagine that you are an artist ready to paint a beautiful picture of health and long life. So far, we have provided the basics of how to paint the picture. *The CR Way* Foods to Choose provides you with the canvas, paint, brush, and easel—the tools necessary to use your newfound knowledge to create the most striking picture of health imaginable. Now it is up to you to select what you are going to eat, design your dishes, map out your meals, and get as creative as you want to.

The CR Way offers an abundance of choices, and just as we make each calorie count by choosing foods that are packed with vital nutrients, we combine foods and seasonings to make each bite delicious.

FOODS TO CHOOSE AND ENJOY ON *THE CR WAY*

The following foods make our list for a variety of reasons. Most are nutrient-dense and are classified low on the Glycemic Index. Many may prevent cancers from forming. Some lower the amount of cholesterol circulating in the bloodstream. And all of them are delicious.

ANIMAL PROTEIN THAT INCLUDES
SOME GOOD FAT

Salmon with no salt added—Alaskan, wild—canned, fresh,
   or frozen
Sardines with no oil added—canned, fresh, or frozen
Tuna with no oil added—canned, fresh, or frozen

GOOD FAT SOURCES

Almonds
Avocados
Grapeseed oil
Hazelnuts
Olive oil, extra virgin (EVO)
Pecans
Pistachios
Walnuts

BEANS—
LARGELY COMPLEX CARBOHYDRATES
WITH SOME PROTEIN

Adzuki beans
Anasazi beans
Baby limas
Black-eyed peas
Black turtle beans
Garbanzo beans (chickpeas)
   Chana dal (split baby chickpeas, which have the lowest GI
      of any bean)
Lentils, red or green

Mung beans
Pinto beans
Soybeans

VEGGIES WITH LOW GI RANKING

Brassica—The broccoli group

Bok choy (Chinese cabbage)
Broccoli
Brussels sprouts
Cabbage
Cauliflower
Chard, Swiss and red
Collard greens
Kale

Kohlrabi
Mustard greens
Parsley
Radishes, including red,
    black, and white (daikon)
Spinach
Turnip
Turnip greens

Additional leaves
Arugula
Romaine lettuce

Bulbs
Garlic
Leeks
Onions

Mushrooms
Maitake
Portabella
Shiitake

Roots
  Burdock
  Celery root (celeriac, celery knob)

Fruit of the plants
  Eggplant
  Cucumber
  Peppers—red, green, orange, purple, yellow
  Summer squash
  Tomato
  Zucchini

VEGGIES WITH MEDIUM GI RANKING

Roots and tubers
  Beets
  Carrots
  Sweet potatoes

Squash
  Butternut squash
  Pumpkin

Beans
  Green peas

GRAINS

  Barley
  Bread, Sprouted-grain
  Quinoa
  Wild rice

Barley—We like both hulled, which has been processed so minimally to remove the outer chaff that it is still considered a whole grain, and hull-less (a different species that naturally has no hull, often labeled "hulless") for texture. We love it and eat large amounts of it, as you'll see in our recipes. If you haven't eaten barley before, you may want to start out with small amounts and increase your intake slowly because of its cathartic effect, which causes bowel activity. You may also prefer to start out with pearled barley, which is processed considerably more for fiber removal, but is still low glycemic and still tastes good.

Quinoa—Lovely and light, quinoa looks like a close relative of couscous, but it's not couscous. Like couscous, though, it's also not a grain. It's actually a seed but is widely regarded as a grain—ever since its days as the "gold" of the ancient Incas. What really matters is its nutrient content. Compared to other vegetable foods, quinoa is very high in the B vitamins, minerals, and amino acids.

Wild Rice—A nutty flavor and crunchy texture characterize this grain (it is not a rice), which is still gathered wild. Versatile and fun, it works in everything from casseroles to desserts, from bread or cereal to a side dish. It has a moderate GI ranking and is rich in several vitamins and minerals.

Bread—Spouted-grain—The GI ranking of most breads is too high and the nutrient content too low to bring along on *The CR Way*, but sprouted-grain breads provide a whole different experience. The best sprouted-grain breads are made with all three layers of the grain—including the outer layer, the internal germ, and the endosperm. This results in a wonderfully nutrient-dense food that is loaded with vitamins, minerals, and phytochemicals.

Sprouting the grains avoids the need for flour. Unpublished research shows that these breads have a moderate effect on the glucose level. It is also reported that sprouted-grain bread is more easily digested and that people with wheat intolerance find that they can digest sprouted grain without difficulty.

The ones we know and use:
Ezekiel 4:9, by Food for Life
Ezekiel 4:9, low sodium, by Food for Life
Genesis 2:29, by Food for Life, seedier, grainier

FRUIT

All fruit should be eaten in whole pieces without any added sweetener. Fruit juice, except as noted below, has glycemic rankings that are too high.

Apricots
Blackberries
Blueberries
Cantaloupe (This is a great food: Canteloupe has good nutrients and moderate glycemic effect. But cases have been reported of dangerous microbes on the skin being carried into the fruit during cutting. Our solution is to thoroughly rinse the melon under running water, peel it, cut the fruit with a clean knife and blanch it for 30 seconds in boiling water.)

Cranberries	Peaches
Kiwi	Raspberries
Lemon	Strawberries
Orange	Tangerines

WHOLE FRUIT OR MODERATE SERVING OF JUICE

Cranberries

Lime

Lemon (We have come to really appreciate lemon and lime
juices. Mixed with olive oil, either makes the base of
sauces that we often use several times a day—with gusto.
And to reduce oxidation of freshly cooked vegetables we
sprinkle them with these zesty juices.)

SPICES AND HERBS

Season foods with enhancing herbs and spices rather than with salt,
pepper, butter, and sugar.

Basil	Ginger
Bay leaf	Marjoram
Cardamom	Mustard seed
Chives	Oregano
Cilantro	Parsley
Cloves	Rosemary
Cumin	Tarragon
Dill	Turmeric
Garlic, ground or chopped	

HERBAL TEAS

Burdock

Dandelion

Ginger

Peppermint

Rosemary

FIBER

Besides all the fiber we get in the rest of our food, whole and ground flaxseeds provide an enjoyable, crunchy fiber addition to most of the vegetables, beans, and grains listed here.

FOODS FOR A HEALTHY HEART

Food choices make a huge difference in heart and artery health.

Avoid Bad Fats.

Purge your diet of all bad fats, including:

- Partially hydrogenated (trans) fats, such as shortening and margarine
- Saturated fat, such as in meats, some dairy products, and tropical oils like palm and coconut

Most trans fat is created when manufacturers turn liquid oils into more solid fats like shortening and margarine. Any food that has partially hydrogenated fat in it has the potential to do real damage to your arteries.

Study after study link saturated fat to increased risk for heart disease as well as diabetes and cancer. And even small amounts show up in testing. We look for 5 grams or less, and preferably zero gram of saturated fat in a serving of food. Completely avoid foods that are especially high in saturated fats.

UNFRIENDLY FATS

FATS THAT RAISE CHOLESTEROL	SOURCES	EXAMPLES
Dietary cholesterol	Foods from animals	Dairy products; meats, especially organ meats (heart, etc.)
Saturated fats	Foods from animals	Meats, lard, and whole-fat dairy products
	Foods from plants	Chocolate, cocoa butter
	Candy	Candies that contain stearic or palmitic acid
Trans fats (partially hydrogenated vegetable oils)	Processed foods	Cookies, crackers, cakes, French fries, fried onion rings, donuts
Tropical oils	Certain plant oils	Palm, palm kernel and coconut oils

Don't Cook Fat. Sorry!

Replace unhealthy fats with healthy ones, such as olive or grapeseed oil. Since cooking fats can produce carcinogens, always add oil to food only *after* it is cooked. Our principal cooking method is boiling foods with water or broth over a low or medium heat. This kills microbes while retaining as much nutrient value as possible.

Add Some Good Fat to Every Meal

For decades now, people have heard that fat is bad, so they think it is healthy to choose foods that are labeled "fat-free." Eating foods that have no trans fat and little saturated fat is smart, but eating carbohydrates without any fat at all is a bad idea. When you eat carbs without fat, the body converts part of them to fats known as triglycerides, which, when elevated, are a risk factor for heart disease and atherosclerosis. Fat-free meals actually *increase* the amount of bad fat in your bloodstream, so always include some good-quality fat with every meal. For delicious healthy fat sources, see page 150.

Fruits and Vegetables

With all the recommendations to eat a heart-friendly diet that includes more fruits and vegetables, you might have expected that *The CR Way* would include all fruits. However, we discriminate against fruits if they are high in fructose, which is linked to an increased risk of AGE (Advanced Glycation Endproducts), that nasty combination of proteins and glucose or fats associated with atherosclerosis and heart disease, along with a whole host of other unwelcome conditions. High fructose consumption in beverages has been linked to increased heart disease risk by raising blood levels of cholesterol and triglycerides.

HEART-HEALTHY FRUITS TO CHOOSE

Blackberries
Blueberries
Cranberries
Raspberries
Strawberries

Salt (Sodium Chloride)

SODIUM LABELING

Although labels vary in the terms they use to describe the amount of salt in a product, here is a rough guide:

SODIUM FREE
Less than 5 mg per serving

VERY LOW SODIUM
35 mg or less per serving

LOW SODIUM
140 mg or less per serving

REDUCED SODIUM
75 percent reduction in sodium content from original product

UNSALTED, NO SALT ADDED, WITHOUT ADDED SALT
Processed without salt when salt normally would be used in processing

You may think that because CR triggers such low blood pressure, eating salt is okay. Actually, reducing salt in the diet is one way calorie restrictors keep their blood pressure low. Decreasing your salt intake is a dietary choice that will allow you to take advantage of CR's longevity effects. A little salt for flavor is fine but remember: everything in moderation. Besides, as you experiment with spices and herbs, you will probably find that you want the salt less.

A completely sodium-free diet, in fact, may put you in danger of irregular heartbeat. A warning sign that salt avoidance has gone too far is muscle cramps, especially in your legs. If you get cramps, try *gradually* increasing your sodium intake until the cramps go away.

Many Foods Fight Cancer

CANCER-FIGHTING FOODS	CANCER-FIGHTING EFFECTS
Fats	
Fish and ground flaxseed Omega-3 essential fatty acids	Reduce likelihood of colon cancer and prostate cancer
Olive oil, extra virgin (EVO)	EVO's main fatty acid, oleic acid, is antioncogenic.
Walnuts	Antioxidant and anticarcinogenic effects
Fruit	
Black raspberries	Preventative effect against oral and esophageal cancers
Blueberries	Kill colon and prostate cancer cells in lab studies
Cranberries	Effective against breast, colon, and prostate cancer cells in research studies
Lemons	Possible prevention of thyroid cancer in humans
	Effectively fight colon and liver cancer in lab animals
	Effectively fight breast, prostate, liver, and colon cancer cell lines in laboratory studies
Limes	Effectively fight breast cancer cell lines in the lab
Raspberries	Effective against liver cancer cells in research studies
Strawberries	Effective against esophageal cancer in lab animals

Grains

Barley — Contains high concentration of beta-glucan fiber, which suppresses tumor growth

Legumes

Black beans — Reduce colon cancer

Soybeans — Prevent prostate cancer

Lentils and lentil soup, cooked from dried beans — Reduce colorectal cancer recurrence

Mushrooms

Shiitake and maitake — Contain high concentration of beta-glucan fiber, which suppress tumor growth

Vegetables

Brassicas, the broccoli bunch — Prevent cancer more effectively than an overall increase in fruits and vegetables

Arugula   Collard greens

Bok choy   Kale

Broccoli   Kohlrabi — Prevent thyroid, breast, lung, and prostate cancers. Enhance treatment of lung, stomach, colorectal, oral, esophageal, Tomatoes pancreatic, bladder, and cervical cancers

Brussels sprouts   Mustard greens

Cabbages   Radish

Cauliflower   Turnip

Bell peppers — Capsiates in peppers target a variety of pathways involved in cancer development and inflammation

Garlic, garlic powder — Prevent cancer, especially liver and colon cancers

| Cloves, ginger, cumin, basil, and rosemary | Prevent and treat a variety of inflammatory diseases, including cancer, in laboratory animals |

Once you regularly experience the flavors, textures, aromas, and health benefits from the Foods to Choose, you will likely be on *The CR Way* for the rest of your life.

10

MENUS AND RECIPES

We keep several things in mind when preparing our food: time constraints, family preferences, individual tastes, and the most important—making meals that will provide the maximum benefit from CR.

Time

The CR Way is an ideal lifestyle for our fast-paced society. We all lead busy lives and most of us simply don't have time to use elaborate recipes. So everything you find here is easy—requiring minimal preparation time. For example, we don't cook every day. Our strategy is to use a big soup pot and make large amounts—beans, veggies, barley—whatever. We use some the day we cook, refrigerate some, and freeze the rest so that food is ready for several days.

Family

You needn't feel isolated from the family dinner table while practicing CR. Rather, adapting CR meals around your family preferences is easy because the staples of healthful, balanced meals are already on the Foods to Choose list. Meals can be prepared for the entire family to share or as individual servings. For children who are not joining you in CR, you can build on the recipes here, adding whatever they love to the menu and still enjoy mealtime together as a family.

Individual Tastes

You can and should, of course, experiment with food combinations that appeal to you. Any of these recipes can be adapted to suit your personal preferences—perhaps you're having people over to dinner or wish to create a special-occasion meal. Your choices are boundless, limited only by your imagination.

Food Selection to Maximize CR Benefits

All foods and recipes are selected with these criteria in mind:

- Nutrient density
  - High nutrient content per calorie
  - Moderate to low Glycemic Index rankings
- Carbohydrate-Protein-Fat (CPF) ratio that emphasizes complex carbs and includes good fats
- Organic ingredients to reduce unwanted agricultural chemicals from nonorganic pesticides, herbicides, fertilizers, and hormones (see page 117, Chapter 7; "Cancer Prevention")
- Low AGE levels (see Advanced Glycation Endproducts, page 68, Chapter 4, "Glucose Control")
- And, of course: satisfying and flavorful

Once you get the hang of CR, you can use the Foods to Choose guide to create your own meal options. Just be sure to use your glucose meter to ensure that your choices are helping you keep glucose levels where you want them.

SAMPLE MEAL PLANS

The easiest way to show you how to plan a CR meal is with a meal plan that's usable at any level of caloric reduction. You would vary only the amounts of the dishes prepared. This also demonstrates how easily you can share the same food preparation with others who eat with different intentions. But first, let's see what's on the menu. (Recipe section begin. on page 179.)

THE CR WAY MENU OF THE DAY

Tease Meal
Peppers and Onions Tease

Breakfast Main Meal
Must-Have Mung Beans dressed with
organic extra virgin olive oil and lemon juice
Wheat Berry Cereal
Lemon-Ginger Sweet Potatoes, drizzled with
organic extra virgin olive oil

Lunch
Curried Lima Beans
Potluck Vegetable Soup, served over
Savory Barley or sprouted-grain bread with organic extra virgin olive oil
Kohlrabi and Spinach, served with or over
Sprouted-grain bread or Savory Barley
English Walnuts

Dinner
Mushroom Magic Soup, served with or over

Sprouted-grain bread or Savory Barley
drizzled with organic extra virgin olive oil
Lemon-Ginger Sweet Potatoes, drizzled with organic extra virgin olive oil
English Walnuts

REDUCTION LEVELS

The following tables provide sample meals for the amounts of CR described on page 46, Chapter 3; "CR As You Like It." The meals are intended as examples—you may not be of the indicated height, age, or activity level, but these models show you the pattern, and from there you can determine where you would like to start.

An important feature that shows up in our meal plan analyses is the Carbohydrate-Protein-Fat (CPF) ratio. Calculating from the DRI tables, an optimal CPF ratio is 60 percent carbs to 10 percent to 15 percent protein to 25 percent to 30 percent fat. All three are essential to life. Since too much protein can overstimulate growth-related hormones and it has been known for a long time that too much fat isn't good for our health, we pay attention to the balance.

Following are analyses of sample meals that three men and three women enjoyed from the preceding menu. Each of them is reducing calorie intake by 5 percent, 10 percent to 15 percent, or 20 percent. Each of them enjoys a breakfast, lunch, and dinner from the menu. So take a look at the analyses—quite easy to do with nutritional software like NutriBase, which generated these data and which helps us make our nutritional decisions.

BREAKFAST MEAL PLAN AT 5%, 10% TO 15%, AND 20% REDUCTION LEVELS FOR WOMEN WHO NORMALLY EAT 2000 CALORIES PER DAY (45 YEARS OLD, MEDIUM BUILD, MODERATELY ACTIVE)

DAILY CALORIE INTAKE GOALS:	5% REDUCTION 1900			10% TO 15% REDUCTION 1700–1800			20% REDUCTION 1600		
	Serving size in grams	Conventional equivalent	Calories	Serving size in grams	Conventional equivalent	Calories	Serving size in grams	Conventional equivalent	Calories
Peppers and Onions Tease	129	1/2 cup	120	129	1/2 cup	120	129	1/2 cup	120
Must-Have Mung Beans	250	1 cup (heaping)	243	220	1 cup	214	195	1 cup (scant)	190
Lemon-Ginger Sweet Potatoes	80	1/3 cup	61	65	1/4 cup	49	65	1/4 cup	49
Olive oil	13	1 tbsp.	117	11	1 1/2 tsp.	99	9	1 3/4 tsp.	81
Lemon juice	20	4 tsp.	5	20	4 tsp.	5	18	4 tsp.	5

(continued)

BREAKFAST MEAL PLAN AT 5%, 10% TO 15%, AND 20% REDUCTION LEVELS FOR *WOMEN* WHO NORMALLY EAT 2000 CALORIES PER DAY (45 YEARS OLD, MEDIUM BUILD, MODERATELY ACTIVE)

DAILY CALORIE INTAKE GOALS:	5% REDUCTION 1900			10% TO 15% REDUCTION 1700–1800			20% REDUCTION 1600		
	Serving size in grams	Conventional equivalent	Calories	Serving size in grams	Conventional equivalent	Calories	Serving size in grams	Conventional equivalent	Calories
Wheat Berry Cereal	365	1½ cups	357	303	1⅓ cups	296	325	1½ (scant) cups	318
Total breakfast calories			903			783			763
Breakfast CPF ratio		60-13-27			59-13-29			61-13-26	

(continued)

BREAKFAST MEAL PLAN AT 5%, 10% TO 15%, AND 20% REDUCTION LEVELS FOR *MEN* WHO NORMALLY EAT 2500 CALORIES PER DAY (45 YEARS OLD, MEDIUM BUILD, MODERATELY ACTIVE)

DAILY CALORIE INTAKE GOALS:	5% REDUCTION 2375			10% TO 15% REDUCTION 2125–2250			20% REDUCTION 2000		
	Serving size in grams	Conventional equivalent	Calories	Serving size in grams	Conventional equivalent	Calories	Serving size in grams	Conventional equivalent	Calories
Peppers and Onions Tease	129	1 serving	120	129	1 serving	120	129	1 serving	120
Must-Have Mung Beans	300	1⅓ cups	292	300	1⅓ cups	292	276	1 cup (heaping)	269
Lemon–Ginger Sweet Potatoes	80	⅓ cup	61	80	⅓ cup	61	80	⅓ cup	61
Olive oil	15	1 tbsp.	135	15	1 tbsp.	135	15	1 tbsp.	135

(continued)

BREAKFAST MEAL PLAN AT 5%, 10% TO 15%, AND 20% REDUCTION LEVELS
FOR *MEN* WHO NORMALLY EAT 2500 CALORIES PER DAY
(45 YEARS OLD, MEDIUM BUILD, MODERATELY ACTIVE)

DAILY CALORIE INTAKE GOALS:	5% REDUCTION 2375			10% TO 15% REDUCTION 2125–2250			20% REDUCTION 2000		
	Serving size in grams	Conventional equivalent	Calories	Serving size in grams	Conventional equivalent	Calories	Serving size in grams	Conventional equivalent	Calories
Lemon juice	30	2 tsp.	8	30	2 tsp.	8	24	1½ tsp.	6
Wheat Berry Cereal	400	1¾ cups	391	378	1½ cups	369	376	1½ cups	369
Total breakfast calories			1007			985			960
Breakfast CPF ratio		60-13-27			60-13-27			60-12-28	

LUNCH MEAL PLAN AT 5%, 10% TO 15%, AND 20% REDUCTION LEVELS FOR *WOMEN* WHO NORMALLY EAT 2000 CALORIES PER DAY (45 YEARS OLD, MEDIUM BUILD, MODERATELY ACTIVE)

DAILY CALORIE INTAKE GOALS:	5% REDUCTION 1900			10% TO 15% REDUCTION 1700–1800			20% REDUCTION 1600		
	Serving size in grams	Conventional equivalent	Calories	Serving size in grams	Conventional equivalent	Calories	Serving size in grams	Conventional equivalent	Calories
Curried Lima Beans	125	1/2 cup (rounded)	111	150	1/2 cup (heaping)	133	75	1/3 cup	66
Potluck Vegetable Soup Served with	263	1 cup (rounded)	132	300	1 1/3 cups	107	345	1 1/2 cups	173
Sprouted-grain bread with	17	1/2 slice	40	17	1/2 slice	40	34	1 slice	80
Olive oil	12	2.5 tsp.	106	9	1 3/4 tsp.	81	8	1 2/3 tsp.	72
Savory Barley	175	3/4 cup	155	172	3/4 cup	152			

(continued)

(continued)

LUNCH MEAL PLAN AT 5%, 10% TO 15%, AND 20% REDUCTION LEVELS FOR *WOMEN* WHO NORMALLY EAT 2000 CALORIES PER DAY (45 YEARS OLD, MEDIUM BUILD, MODERATELY ACTIVE)

DAILY CALORIE INTAKE GOALS:	5% REDUCTION 1900			10% TO 15% REDUCTION 1700–1800			20% REDUCTION 1600		
	Serving size in grams	Conventional equivalent	Calories	Serving size in grams	Conventional equivalent	Calories	Serving size in grams	Conventional equivalent	Calories
Kohlrabi and Spinach	135	½ cup (rounded)	34	135	½ cup (rounded)	34	150	½ cup (heaping)	38
Walnuts, English Dried and crushed	5	1 tsp.	33	8	1 2/3 tsp.	52	4		26
Total lunch calories			607			599			455
CPF ratio, Lunch		60-13-27			=62-13-25			60-16-24	

LUNCH MEAL PLAN 5%, 10% TO 15%, AND 20% REDUCTION LEVELS FOR *MEN* WHO NORMALLY EAT 2500 CALORIES PER DAY (45 YEARS OLD, MEDIUM BUILD, MODERATELY ACTIVE)

DAILY CALORIE INTAKE GOALS:	5% REDUCTION 2375			10% TO 15% REDUCTION 2125–2250			20% REDUCTION 2000		
	Serving size in grams	Conventional equivalent	Calories	Serving size in grams	Conventional equivalent	Calories	Serving Size in grams	Conventional equivalent	Calories
Curried Lima Beans				150	⅔ cup	133	120	½ cup	106
Potluck Vegetable Soup Served with	300	1⅓ cup	150	200	¾ cup (heaping)	100	230	1 cup	115
Sprouted-grain bread Drizzled with	34	1 slice	80	17	½ slice	40	17	½ slice	40
Olive oil, extra virgin, Organic	12	2½ tsp.	106	11	2¼ tsp. (heaping)	99	10	2 tsp.	88
Kohlrabi and Spinach Garnished with	250	1 cup	64	135	½ cup (heaping)	34	135	½ cup	34
Walnuts, English Dried, crushed	15	3 tsp.	98	5	1 tsp.	33	5	1 tsp.	33

(continued)

(continued)

LUNCH MEAL PLAN 5%, 10% TO 15%, AND 20% REDUCTION LEVELS FOR *MEN* WHO NORMALLY EAT 2500 CALORIES PER DAY (45 YEARS OLD, MEDIUM BUILD, MODERATELY ACTIVE)

DAILY CALORIE INTAKE GOALS:	5% REDUCTION 2375			10% TO 15% REDUCTION 2125–2250			20% REDUCTION 2000		
	Serving size in grams	Conventional equivalent	Calories	Serving size in grams	Conventional equivalent	Calories	Serving Size in grams	Conventional equivalent	Calories
Savory Barley	380	1²/₃ cups	328	350	1¹/₂ cup	302	230	1 cup	199
Total lunch calories			827		740				616
Lunch CPF ratio			60-12-28			63-12-25			59-13-28

DINNER MEAL PLAN AT 5%, 10% TO 15%, AND 20% REDUCTION LEVELS FOR *WOMEN* WHO NORMALLY EAT 2000 CALORIES PER DAY (45 YEARS OLD, MEDIUM BUILD, MODERATELY ACTIVE)

DAILY CALORIE INTAKE GOALS:	5% REDUCTION 1900			10% TO 15% REDUCTION 1700–1800			20% REDUCTION 1600		
	Serving size in grams	Conventional equivalent	Calories	Serving size in grams	Conventional equivalent	Calories	Serving size in grams	Conventional equivalent	Calories
Mushroom Magic Soup	205	3/4 cup (heaping)	71	410	1 3/4 cups	143	308	1 1/2 cups	107
Sprouted-grain bread with	34	1 slice	80	34	1 slice	80			
Olive oil, extra virgin, Organic	10 1/2	2 1/2 tsp.	94	11	2 1/3 tsp.	99	10	2 tsp.	90
Lemon–Ginger Sweet Potatoes	150	2/3 cup	155	100	1/2 cup (scant)	103	50	1/4 cup (scant)	52
Savory Barley							150	2/3 cup	133

(continued)

(*continued*)

DINNER MEAL PLAN AT 5%, 10% TO 15%, AND 20% REDUCTION LEVELS
FOR *WOMEN* WHO NORMALLY EAT 2000 CALORIES PER DAY
(45 YEARS OLD, MEDIUM BUILD, MODERATELY ACTIVE)

DAILY CALORIE INTAKE GOALS:	5% REDUCTION 1900		10% TO 15% REDUCTION 1700–1800		20% REDUCTION 1600	
	CPF Ratio	Calories	CPF Ratio	Calories	CPF Ratio	Calories
Total Dinner Intake		400		425		382
Whole Day Intake		1902		1804		1603
Dinner	59-13-28		60-12-28		60-13-27	
Whole Day	60-14-26		61-13-27		60-14-24	

DINNER MEAL PLAN AT 5%, 10% TO 15%, AND 20% REDUCTION LEVELS FOR MEN WHO ARE NORMALLY EATING 2500 CALORIES PER DAY (45 YEARS OLD, MEDIUM BUILD, MODERATELY ACTIVE)

DAILY CALORIE INTAKE GOALS:	5% REDUCTION 2375			10% TO 15% REDUCTION 2125–2250			20% REDUCTION 2000		
	Serving in grams	Conventional equivalent	Calories	Serving in grams	Conventional equivalent	Calories	Serving in grams	Conventional equivalent	Calories
Mushroom Magic Soup	250	1 cup	119	616	2⅔ cups	214	345	1 cup	164
Sprouted-grain bread with	17	½ slice	40				34	1 slice	80
Olive oil (EVO)	12	2½ tsp.	108	6	1¼ tsp.	54	10	2 tsp.	88
Lemon–Ginger Sweet Potatoes	230	1 cup	237	100	½ cup (scant)	76	125	½ cup	95
Walnuts, English Dried, crushed	5	1 tsp.	33	7	1½ tsp.	46			

(continued)

(continued)

DINNER MEAL PLAN AT 5%, 10% TO 15%, AND 20% REDUCTION LEVELS FOR MEN WHO ARE NORMALLY EATING 2500 CALORIES PER DAY (45 YEARS OLD, MEDIUM BUILD, MODERATELY ACTIVE)

DAILY CALORIE INTAKE GOALS:	5% REDUCTION 1900			10% TO 15% REDUCTION 1700–1800			20% REDUCTION 1600		
	Serving in grams	Conventional equivalent	Calories	Serving in grams	Conventional equivalent	Calories	Serving in grams	Conventional equivalent	Calories
Average pre-CR daily intake			2500			2500			2500
Reduced daily intake goal			2375			2125–2250			2000
Whole day calorie intake			2378			2253			2000
Total dinner calories			537			497			385
Dinner CPF ratio			63-9-28			63-13-24			59-13-27
Whole day CPF ratio			62-11-27			62-13-25			60-13-28

RECIPES

As you review the meal plans, you will probably want to look at the recipes. The starred recipes in the meal plans and some others that we especially like are detailed in the following pages. Because some of the ingredients are not always easy to find, we've included some brand names.

We have developed these recipes over the years that we've been on *The CR Way*. They work for us, and we hope that they help you get started—after which you will develop your own versions and new creations. As you craft new scrumptious, nutritious recipes, we hope you will share them with us at our Web site: www .LivingTheCRWay.com.

Nutritional Analysis

The most plentiful nutritive components of each recipe are highlighted in a nutrient box, which includes, whenever possible, information per serving that would be helpful in following *The CR Way* recommendations. For example, you will see the amounts of omega-3 and omega-6 fatty acids in salmon, walnuts, and a few other sources that are *CR Way* staples.

The nutritional analysis of the recipes was done by NutriBase, the software we use for dietary tracking. The basis for the nutritional information in each food comes primarily from the U.S. Department of Agriculture. Information on foods that are not in databases included in NutriBase, like Tuscan tomatoes, comes from the manufacturers.

Type of sugar matters

To minimize AGE formation—knowing what kind of sugar you take into your body is important, so you will find measures of fructose, which is more prone to the formation of AGE.

Phytochemicals

The presence of phytosterols gives a hint of the beneficial phytochemicals in a particular food. Phytochemical analysis is in its infancy, and we hope to draw attention to its importance.

Vitamin A

Vitamin A is expressed in RAE, or Retinol Activity Equivalents. Carotenoids are also listed. According to NutriBase, the carotenoids in the analysis do not contribute much to actual vitamin A activity, but they play important roles as antioxidants and may reduce risks of cancer and other diseases. So, for the ultimate disease protection, knowing this information is important.

Wheat berries

Detailed nutritional analysis from the USDA is not yet available for wheat berries. However, we were able to benefit from a very thorough analysis available from the Danish Food Composition Databank of Denmark's National Food Institute.

CR WAY RECIPES—EASY AND DELICIOUS

VEGGIE DISHES

You have no doubt noticed that vegetables are a mainstay of *The CR Way*. And why not? They can provide excellent nutrition from complex carbohydrates without the drawbacks of foods that are higher in fats and proteins. We need all three, of course, and veggies help us keep the balance weighted in favor of complex carbs.

EASY VEGGIES

Vegetables with low-glycemic effect are what we look for on *The CR Way*. This is just one of many vegetable dishes that can be prepared and used at once, or saved for later use on its own or as an ingredient in other dishes. It can be served as a light soup, or over Savory Barley (recipe on page 205-206) or sprouted-grain bread (description, page 153, Chapter 9). Or the veggies can be strained, with the broth saved for later use, and the vegetables served as a side dish. In all these cases, dressing with extra virgin olive oil and lemon juice improves the flavor and the nutrition. Using frozen vegetables gives this dish its name. Low-glycemic, nutrient-dense vegetables are available in various frozen assortments—for example, broccoli, cauliflower, carrot, green beans, and bell peppers in a variety of colors.

Makes four 5-ounce+ (150 gm.) servings with some left for tease meals

  1 bay leaf
  1 medium-large onion (240 gm)
  6 medium garlic cloves (36 gm)
  1 16-ounce package of frozen low-glycemic veggies or equivalent combination

Dressing

  1½ teaspoons (7 gm) extra virgin olive oil per serving
  1 tablespoon lemon juice

Easy Veggies	
Calories:	42
Protein (g):	1.08
Carbohydrates (g):	8.82
Sugars (g):	3.32
Glucose (g):	0.80
Fructose (g):	0.49
Dietary Fiber (g):	3.12
Fat (g):	0.25
Saturated Fat (g):	0.05
Phytosterols (mg):	5.64
Vit-A (mcg_RAE):	161.05
Carotene, beta (mcg):	1579.43
Carotene, alpha (mcg):	711.10
Lycopene (mcg):	0.38
Lutein+zeaxanthin (mcg):	153.90
Total Folate (mcg):	24.34
Vit-C (mg):	24.08
Vit-K (mcg):	8
Calcium (mg):	34
Magnesium (mg):	12.21
Phosphorus (mg):	27.68
Potassium (mg):	149.35
Sodium (mg):	25.69

1. Bring a quart of water with bay leaf, onion, and garlic to a boil.

2. Boil over medium heat for about 5 minutes, depending on the onion's pungency.

3. Add the vegetables, return to a boil over medium heat till the vegetables start to simmer.

4. Dish, dress, and serve.

TURNIP AND EDAMAME

Serving Suggestions

- Serve as soup.
- Drain and serve as vegetable dish.
- Serve soup, with or over Savory Barley or sprouted-grain bread.

Makes four 5-ounce+ (150gm) servings with some left for tease meals

1 large bay leaf

1 medium onion (240gm), ½-inch diced

6 medium garlic cloves, cut in half or as desired

1 medium turnip (180gm), cut into ¾-inch pieces

1 pound frozen organic edamame, blanched, shelled

½ teaspoon curry powder, or to taste

Turnip and Edamame	
Calories:	159.95
Protein (g):	12.08
Carbohydrates (g):	15.65
Sugars (g):	4.31
Glucose (g):	0.46
Fructose (g):	0.27
Dietary Fiber (g):	4.38
Fat (g):	5.77
Saturated Fat (g):	1.15
Polyunsaturated Fat (g):	0.04
Phytosterols (mg):	5.48
Vit-B5 Pantothenic Acid (mg):	0.10
Vit-B6 Pyridoxine (mg):	0.11
Vit-C (mg):	21.81
Calcium (mg):	134.51
Magnesium (mg):	6.70
Phosphorus (mg):	19.94
Potassium (mg):	102.09
Sodium (mg):	30.23
Iron (mg):	2.30
Manganese (mg):	0.14
Selenium (mcg):	0.88

1. Place 2 cups water in a pot; add the bay leaf, onion, and garlic. Bring to a boil.

2. Boil gently, uncovered, 4 to 5 minutes.

3. Add the turnip. Continue to boil on medium heat for 3 minutes.

4. Add the edamame. Return to a boil and cook on low heat for 5 to 6 minutes, or until tender.

5. Add the curry powder and stir to distribute evenly.

6. Remove the bay leaf before serving.

CILANTRO'D VEGGIES

Cilantro is the leaves (and stems) of the coriander plant. In ancient times, it was among the spices considered to have aphrodisiac effects. We make no claims, except that it's reminiscent of citrus and parsley and is a good addition to this and other vegetable dishes. To get the maximum flavor out of this herb, put most of it in the pot to start and add the rest close to the end of the cooking process. Using fresh vegetables in place of frozen will require adding them with the turnip and increasing cooking time until the veggies are just getting tender.

Cilantro'd Veggies	
Calories:	46.57
Protein (g):	2.49
Carbohydrates (g):	9.58
Sugars (g):	4.88
Glucose (g):	0.29
Fructose (g):	0.17
Dietary Fiber (g):	3.17
Fat (g):	0.04
Phytosterols (mg):	4.06
Vit-A IU:	175.69
Vit-C (mg):	24.89
Calcium (mg):	33.85

Serving Suggestions

- Serve alone as soup.
- Serve soup over sprouted-grain bread or Savory Barley.
- Drain and serve over Savory Barley, saving the broth for later use.

Makes four 5-ounce+ (150 gm) servings

1 medium-large onion, ½-inch diced (240 gm)

4 medium garlic cloves, cut in half or as desired (24 gm)

2 teaspoons cilantro, dried

1¼ cups turnip (287 gm), ½-inch diced

1 10-ounce package frozen mixed mushrooms

1 16-ounce package frozen broccoli florets

1 16-ounce package frozen green beans

Dressing for individual servings

1½ teaspoon organic extra virgin olive oil (5 gm)

1 tablespoon lemon juice (14 gm)

1. Add the onion, garlic, and 1½ teaspoons cilantro to 8 cups (2 quarts) water in a pot.

2. Bring to a boil. Boil on medium heat for 2 minutes.

3. Add the turnip and mushrooms. Return to a boil and cook on medium heat for 4 minutes.

4. Add the frozen vegetables and the last ½ teaspoon cilantro. Cook on medium heat until it barely comes to a boil.

5. Dish, dress, and serve.

BASIC BEETS

Serving Suggestion

- Place serving of beets on plate. Drizzle with olive oil and sprinkle with ground clove or cardamom to taste.

Makes two 2½-ounce (73 gm) servings with some left for tease meals

1 teaspoon whole cardamom seed
2 medium beets peeled and cut (see note) or thoroughly scrubbed

Dressing for individual servings

1 teaspoon organic extra virgin olive oil
Small pinch ground cloves
Small pinch ground cardamom

Basic Beets	
Calories:	50.26
Protein (g):	1.13
Carbohydrates (g):	7.38
Sugars (g):	4.73
Dietary Fiber (g):	2.30
Fat (g):	2.11
Saturated Fat (g):	0.30
Polyunsaturated Fat (g):	0.33
Phytosterols (mg):	17.51
Vit-A (mcg_RAE):	1.40
Carotene, beta (mcg):	14.01
Vit-A IU:	23.28
Vit-B1 Thiamine (mg):	0.19
Vit-B2 Riboflavin (mg):	0.20
Vit-B5 Pantothenic Acid (mg):	0.11
Total Folate (mcg):	76.33
Calcium (mg):	12.57
Magnesium (mg):	16.11
Phosphorus (mg):	28.01
Potassium (mg):	231.68
Sodium (mg):	54.79

1. Put whole cardamom seed in 2 to 3 cups water in a pan. Bring water to a boil.

2. Add beets and return to a boil.

3. Boil at medium heat for 8 minutes.

4. Drain and cool.

5. Sprinkle with 1 teaspoon, or amount needed, lemon juice to reduce oxidation.

Note: * Beets cut before cooking will "bleed." We clean and cut them to gain a light beet broth. If you don't want broth, leave beets with an inch or two of stem, scrub them with a vegetable brush and cook as above. Peel should be easy to slip off.

LEMON-GINGER SWEET POTATOES

Sweet potatoes are so delicious that even when prepared simply, they are very satisfying.

Serving Suggestions

This recipe can be used for a tease meal or as a side dish with a main meal.

Makes four 2½-ounce (70 gm) servings with some left for tease meals

1 medium-large sweet potato
(10.5 ounces, 300 grams)
Sprinkle of lemon juice, 1 teaspoon or
more as desired

Dressing for individual servings

- ¼ teaspoon ground ginger, or to taste
- Sprinkling of lemon juice
- 6 gm extra virgin olive oil

1. Peel and ⅓-inch dice the sweet potatoes.

2. Sprinkle with lemon juice to reduce oxidation.

3. Bring 2 cups water to a boil in a saucepan, add the sweet potatoes.

4. Cook at medium boil for 4½ minutes. Drain.

Lemon-Ginger Sweet Potatoes	
Calories:	53.22
Protein (g):	0.96
Carbohydrates (g):	12.41
Sugars (g):	4.02
Glucose (g):	0.38
Fructose (g):	0.30
Dietary Fiber (g):	1.75
Fat (g):	0.10
Saturated Fat (g):	0.03
Vit-A (mcg_RAE):	551.06
Carotene, beta (mcg):	6612.77
Vit-B5 Pantothenic Acid (mg):	0.41
Vit-B6 Tyridoxine (mg):	0.12
Vit-C (mg):	8.96
Tocopherol, Alpha (mg):	0.66
Vit-K (mcg):	1.47
Calcium (mg):	18.91
Magnesium (mg):	12.60
Phosphorus (mg):	22.41
Potassium (mg):	161.05
Sodium (mg):	18.91
Manganese (mg):	0.19

5. Spread the potatoes out on a plate for cooling.

6. Sprinkle with lemon juice to reduce oxidation.

7. Sprinkle with ground ginger for a stronger flavor and to reduce oxidation.

8. Drizzle olive oil for flavor and to help control glucose levels.

SAVORY SPINACH

Serving Suggestions

- Delicious served over sprouted-grain bread or Savory Barley (recipe, pages 205–206).
- This recipe can be used for a tease meal or as a side dish with main meal.

Makes four 3½-ounce servings (100 gm)

  2 10-ounce packages frozen, organic, cut spinach

  1 medium onion (240 gm, 8.5oz)

  6 medium garlic cloves, cut in half or as desired

  1 teaspoon dried rosemary or 2 teaspoons fresh rosemary

1. Add onion, garlic, and rosemary to 2 to 3 cups water in a pan.

2. Bring to a boil.

Savory Spinach	
Calories:	38.61
Protein (g):	2.66
Carbohydrates (g):	7.81
Sugars (g):	1.18
Glucose (g):	0.50
Fructose (g):	0.30
Dietary Fiber (g):	2.21
Fat (g):	0.31
Saturated Fat (g):	0.05
Phytosterols (mg):	3.88
Vit-A IU:	5185.91
Vit-B1 Thiamine (mg):	0.08
Vit-B2 Riboflavin (mg):	0.12
Vit-B3 Niacin (mg):	0.36
Vit-B5 Pantothenic Acid (mg):	0.13
Vit-B6 Pyridoxine (mg):	0.22
Total Folate (mcg):	85.34
Vit-C (mg):	20.10
Calcium (mg):	92.67
Magnesium (mg):	43.12
Phosphorus (mg):	45.20
Potassium (mg):	281.48
Sodium (mg):	51.67
Copper (mg):	0.10
Iron (mg):	1.54
Manganese (mg):	0.65
Selenium (mcg):	2.07

3. Add the spinach. Return to a boil.

4. Cook on medium heat for 5 minutes, or until the spinach is completely thawed, using a fork to separate the spinach. Avoid overcooking.

KOHLRABI AND SPINACH

This very versatile veggie dish can be served in a variety of ways:

- As a side dish
- With sprouted-grain bread
- Over barley

If kohlrabi is not available, use another vegetable with a low or medium Glycemic Index, e.g.:

Turnip	1 medium (120 gm), ½-inch diced
Black radish	1 medium (150 gm), ½-inch diced
Red radishes	¼ to ⅓ pound (120 to 180 gm), ½-inch diced

Makes two 5-ounce+ (150 gm) servings with some left for tease meals

1 small bay leaf

1 teaspoon dried rosemary or 2 teaspoons fresh rosemary

1 medium kohlrabi (120 gm), cut into ½-inch pieces

2 10-ounce packages frozen, organic, cut spinach

Kohlrabi and Spinach	
Calories:	38.77
Protein (g):	3.27
Carbohydrates (g):	6.76
Sugars (g):	1.16
Dietary Fiber (g):	5.42
Fat (g):	0.12
Saturated Fat (g):	0.01
Carotene, beta (mcg):	9.79
Vit-A IU:	7433.14
Vit-C (mg):	49.83
Calcium (mg):	109.57
Phosphorus (mg):	20.46
Potassium (mg):	155.86
Sodium (mg):	169.97
Iron (mg):	1.96

Dressing for individual servings

> 1 teaspoon lemon juice
> ½ teaspoon organic extra virgin olive oil
> 1 teaspoon flaxseeds, whole or ground

1. Bring 1 cup water to a boil in a saucepan with the bay leaf, rosemary, and kohlrabi.

2. Cook for 5 minutes on medium boil.

3. Add the spinach and return to a boil.

4. Use a fork to separate the spinach so it cooks evenly.

5. Remove the bay leaf before serving.

6. Plate, dress, and serve.

PEPPERS AND ONIONS

Serving Suggestions

- As a side dish a with the main meal
- As a *CR Way* Sandwich topping

Makes two 4⅔-ounce (133 gm) servings

> 1 medium onion (240 gm), sliced or ½-inch diced
> 3 garlic cloves, cut in half or as desired
> 1 10-ounce package frozen tricolor bell peppers or 10 ounces fresh bell peppers

Peppers and Onions	
Calories:	29.87
Protein (g):	0.86
Carbohydrates (g):	7.03
Sugars (g):	2.93
Glucose (g):	0.72
Fructose (g):	0.43
Dietary Fiber (g):	1.24
Fat (g):	0.04
Phytosterols (mg):	5.50
Vit-A (mcg_RAE):	16.67
Vit-C (mg):	50.78
Vit-K (mcg):	0.19
Calcium (mg):	20.16
Phosphorus (mg):	14.49
Potassium (mg):	64.83
Sodium (mg):	1.61
Manganese (mg):	0.10
Selenium (mcg):	0.61

1. Bring 2 cups water to a boil. Add the onion and garlic. Boil on low heat 5 to 6 minutes.

2. Add the peppers. Return to a boil, stirring occasionally to ensure evenness of cooking.

3. Remove from the heat immediately upon boiling to prevent overcooking.

CARAWAY CABBAGE

Cabbage is a very versatile vegetable. We offer this recipe not only because it is a favorite but also because it is so easy.

Serving Suggestions

- Serve as soup.
- Serve with or over Savory Barley.
- Serve with or over sprouted-grain bread.
- Drain and serve as a vegetable dish.

Makes four 5-ounce+ (150 gm) servings

1 head red cabbage
2 tablespoons whole caraway seeds
1 bay leaf

1. Separate the cabbage leaves from the heart, rinse and

Caraway Cabbage	
Calories:	57.09
Protein (g):	2.78
Carbohydrates (g):	12.53
Sugars (g):	5.75
Glucose (g):	2.64
Fructose (g):	2.24
Dietary Fiber (g):	4.42
Fat (g):	0.74
Saturated Fat (g):	0.07
Phytosterols (mg):	2.63
Carotene, beta (mcg):	988.43
Lycopene (mcg):	29.52
Lutein+zeaxanthin (mcg):	489.25
Vit-A IU:	1648.06
Total Folate (mcg):	26.73
Vit-C (mg):	84.26
Vit-K (mcg):	55.98
Calcium (mg):	89.81
Magnesium (mg):	32.38
Phosphorus (mg):	63.64
Potassium (mg):	403.04
Sodium (mg):	40.16
Iron (mg):	1.73

vegetable-brush the leaves. Devein the large leaves, break or cut into your preferred bite size.

2. Soak in water for a half hour if the cabbage needs freshening.

3. Put caraway seed, bay leaf, cabbage, and 4 quarts water into a pot.

4. Bring to a boil and boil on medium heat for 6 to 10 minutes.

5. Strain from the broth; retain both for use separately or together.

TEASE MEALS

All tease meals here are individual servings—which can be easily doubled, tripled, etc., as necessary to make a larger meal. Other *CR Way* Sandwiches can also be used effectively as tease meals.

PEPPERS AND ONION TEASE

Makes an individual serving

1 Essential Sandwich (page 225-226)
3 ounces Peppers and Onions (page 189-190)

Place the Essential Sandwich on a plate.
Top with peppers and onions.
Sprinkle additional herbs or spices, to taste

Peppers and Onion Tease	
Calories:	120.0
Protein (g):	4.96
Carbohydrates (g):	12.84
Sugars (g):	3.27
Dietary Fiber (g):	12.39
Fat (g):	6.72
Vit-B1 Thiamine (mg):	0.10
Vit-B2 Riboflavin (mg):	0.70
Vit-B3 Niacin (mg):	1.20
Total Folate (mcg):	12.80
Magnesium (mg):	35.00
Phosphorus (mg):	58.00
Potassium (mg):	172.27
Sodium (mg):	66.79
Iron (mg):	0.36
Zinc (mg):	0.38

LENTIL AND TOMATO TEASE MEAL

This recipe demonstrates the benefit of cooking large enough amounts for you to use now and also later. Having prepared Light Lentils (see pages 199-200), you could use some to create a quick, easy, and beneficial tease meal. Serving immediately is a fine option. If the weather begs for a warm, comforting dish—place the bowl of Lentil and Tomato Tease ingredients—*before* the olive oil and walnuts are added—into a water bath for a few minutes. The heat also increases the blending of these very complementary flavors.

Makes two 5-ounce + (150 gm) servings

½ cup (scant) lentils (100 gm)

½ cup (scant: 100 gm) tomatoes, stewed or canned (no salt added)

3 tablespoons (40 gm) Very Veggie, low-salt organic vegetable cocktail

1 teaspoon (rounded) dried oregano (½ gm), or to taste

Shakes of garlic to taste

2 teaspoons lemon juice (10 gm)

1 teaspoon olive oil (5 gm)

5 or 6 walnut halves (10 gm)

Lentil and Tomato Tease	
Calories:	101.75
Protein (g):	4.99
Carbohydrates (g):	14.16
Sugars (g):	3.41
Dietary Fiber (g):	4.40
Fat (g):	3.02
Saturated Fat (g):	0.41
Monounsaturated Fat (g):	2.11
Polyunsaturated Fat (g):	0.32
Phytosterols (mg):	6.32
Vit-A (mcg_RAE):	53.27
Vit-A IU:	4.89
Vit-B5 Pantothenic Acid (mg):	0.31
Vit-B6 Pyridoxine (mg):	0.11
Total Folate (mcg):	85.85
Vit-C (mg):	11.43
Tocopherol, Alpha (mg):	0.34
Vit-E (IU):	0.61
Calcium (mg):	20.15
Magnesium (mg):	17.81
Phosphorus (mg):	88.91
Potassium (mg):	248.82
Sodium (mg):	4.13
Copper (mg):	0.12
Iron (mg):	1.68
Selenium (mcg):	1.68

1. Place all ingredients in a
   bowl, jar, or ramekin. Stir.

2. Serve or warm in water
   bath first.

SAVORY SPINACH TEASE

Makes an individual serving

3 ounces Savory Spinach (see page
187)
1 Essential Sandwich (see page 225)

Place Essential Sandwich on a plate.
Top with savory spinach.

TUSCAN TOMATO TEASE

Makes an individual serving

1 slice sprouted-grain bread (31 to
41 gm) broken or cut to bite size
1 tablespoon lemon juice (14 gm)
1 ½ teaspoons organic extra virgin olive
oil (7 gm)
3 canned whole tomatoes, drained and sliced (5+ ounces, 150 gm)
1 to 2 tablespoons organic vegetable cocktail if desired to further moisten bread
¼ teaspoon oregano, or to taste

Savory Spinach Tease	
Calories:	125.46
Protein (g):	5.33
Carbohydrates (g):	9.12
Sugars (g):	0.57
Glucose (g):	0.25
Fructose (g):	0.15
Dietary Fiber (g):	12.08
Fat (g):	5.28
Saturated Fat (g):	0.51
Monounsaturated Fat (g):	2.50
Polyunsaturated Fat (g):	0.52
Omega-6 (g):	0.01
Phytosterols (mg):	1.89
Carotene, beta (mcg):	0.13
Lutein+zeaxanthin (mcg):	1.52
Vit-A IU:	4586.52
Vit-B1 Thiamine (mg):	0.09
Vit-B2 Riboflavin (mg):	0.53
Vit-B3 Niacin (mg):	0.93
Total Folate (mcg):	12.10
Vit-C (mg):	15.64
Calcium (mg):	70.15
Magnesium (mg):	28.38
Phosphorus (mg):	52.17
Potassium (mg):	118.42
Sodium (mg):	156.65
Copper (mg):	0.02
Iron (mg):	1.45
Selenium (mcg):	0.55

⅛ teaspoon garlic powder or granules,
    or to taste
Optional:
2 or 3 walnuts halves (depending on
    how much fat you have in your CR
    plan)

Combine all the ingredients in a
dish, ramekin, or jar.
Stir to blend.

Tuscan Tomato Tease	
Calories:	133.25
Protein (g):	4.43
Carbohydrates (g):	12.34
Sugars (g):	5.31
Dietary Fiber (g):	9.73
Fat (g):	5.03
Saturated Fat (g):	0.50
Monounsaturated Fat (g):	2.50
Polyunsaturated Fat (g):	0.50
Vit-A (mcg_RAE):	155.64
Vit-B2 Riboflavin (mg):	0.53
Total Folate (mcg):	9.60
Vit-C (mg):	25.40
Calcium (mg):	28.51
Magnesium (mg):	26.26
Phosphorus (mg):	43.51
Potassium (mg):	122.77
Sodium (mg):	51.33
Iron (mg):	0.45
Zinc (mg):	0.28

LEGUMES AND OTHER PROTEINS

BASIC BEANS

Most beans are rich in soluble fiber, which helps to eliminate cholesterol from the body. Not only are they low in fat, but when combined with grains, beans supply high-quality protein that provides a healthy alternative to meat or other animal protein. Except for lentils and mung beans, all the beans listed in Chapter 9: "Foods to Choose" can be prepared using this recipe. In **general**, the thing that changes is the cooking time. In some instances a special flavor can be achieved with an additional ingredient early in the process.

Beans need to be soaked (marinating with spices and herbs is even nicer) overnight—except lentils and mungs, as they would become too soft. Soaking beans reduces the cooking time, thus possibly reducing AGE (Advanced Glycation Endproducts, see Chapter 4 "Glucose Control") production.

Seasoning Tip: When the recipe calls for whole seeds, keeping ground spices and herbs, eg., cardamom, cumin, garlic, and ginger, as well as oregano leaves, handy will allow you to adjust the flavoring as the beans cook. In general, 1 cup dried beans = about 2 cups cooked (lima beans yield about 1¼ cups) 1 pound dried beans = 2 cups dried beans → 4 cups cooked.

Makes four 5-ounce+ (150 gm) servings

For the marinade

> 1 pound dried beans rinsed, soaked, and drained
>
> 2 teaspoons cardamom seeds
>
> 2 teaspoons cumin seeds
>
> 1 large bay leaf

For cooking

> 2 teaspoons cardamom seeds
>
> 2 teaspoons cumin seeds
>
> 1 large bay leaf
>
> 1 medium onion (240 gm), ½-inch diced
>
> 6 medium garlic cloves (36 gm), chopped, cut in half, or prepared as desired

For the dressing

> 1 teaspoon (5 gm) organic extra virgin olive oil or an amount to match your calorie and fat-intake plan
>
> 2 teaspoons (10 gm) lemon or lime juice or twice the amount of olive oil

Marinade

1. Sort the beans to remove any small stones and broken beans. Fill a large bowl with cold water and rinse the beans

several times until no dirt remains. Drain the beans in a colander. Rinse the bowl and pour the beans into the bowl.

2. Add the cardamom and cumin seeds and the bay leaf.

3. Fill the bowl with water to cover the beans by an inch. Stir. Cover and marinate overnight in the refrigerator.

Cooking

1. Bring 2 quarts water, cardamom seeds, cumin, and the bay leaf, onion, garlic, and beans to a boil in a large pot.

2. Cover and boil on medium heat for 15 to 20 minutes, or until the beans are tender.

3. Remove the bay leaves before serving.

Serving

1. Pour oil and juice over the beans.

2. Stir and serve.

GINGERED MUNG BEANS

This recipe gives these crunchy mungs the added interest of the ginger flavor.

Makes four 5-ounce+ (150gm.) servings

Gingered Mung Beans	
Calories:	150.58
Protein (g):	9.05
Carbohydrates (g):	28.22
Sugars (g):	3.94
Dietary Fiber (g):	10.19
Fat (g):	0.55
Saturated Fat (g):	0.16
Phytosterols (mg):	5.40
Vit-B1 Thiamine (mg):	0.23
Total Folate (mcg):	208
Vit-K (mcg):	3.63
Calcium (mg):	44.78
Magnesium (mg):	65.24
Phosphorus (mg):	140.28
Potassium (mg):	398.30
Copper (mg):	0.23
Iron (mg):	1.90
Selenium (mcg):	3.66
Zinc (mg):	1.16

with some left for tease meals

1 pound mung beans

¼ cup sliced fresh ginger root

1 medium onion (240 gm), ½-inch diced

3 medium garlic cloves (18 gm.), cut in half or prepared as desired

1 large bay leaf

Follow Basic Bean recipe (pages 194–196), marinating the beans with the bay leaf for one hour rather than overnight.

1. Bring two quarts water and ginger root to a boil in a large pot.

2. Boil on a medium heat for ten minutes.

3. Add bay leaf, onion, garlic, and beans to pot and bring back to the boil.

4. Cover and boil on medium heat for fifteen to twenty minutes or until beans are tender.

5. Dish and serve alone or with or over Savory Barley or sprouted-grain bread.

MUST-HAVE MUNG BEANS

1. Follow the Basic Beans recipe, (pages 194–196) marinating beans in the

Must-Have Mung Beans	
Calories:	146.00
Protein (g):	9.03
Carbohydrates (g):	27.71
Sugars (g):	3.55
Glucose (g):	0.53
Fructose (g):	0.31
Dietary Fiber (g):	9.32
Fat (g):	0.53
Saturated Fat (g):	0.15
Phytosterols (mg):	4.58
Vit-B5 Pantothenic Acid (mg):	0.56
Vit-B6 Pyridoxine (mg):	0.22
Total Folate (mcg):	187.56
Vit-C (mg):	5.33
Tocopherol, Alpha (mg):	0.18
Vit-K (mcg):	3.37
Calcium (mg):	53.33
Magnesium (mg):	60.48
Phosphorus (mg):	137.15
Potassium (mg):	385.89
Copper (mg):	0.22
Iron (mg):	1.83
Manganese (mg):	0.54
Selenium (mcg):	4.34
Zinc (mg):	1.13

refrigerator for 1 hour rather than overnight.

2. Adjust flavoring with garlic powder or granules and ground cumin, cardomom, and ginger, to taste.

3. Place 150- to 200-gram servings in bowls.

4. Dress with a little of the cooking broth and serve with sprouted-grain bread.

ADZUKI CHILI

Adzuki beans are a hard, dark, red bean variety. They are a good source of many nutrients. Being low in fat, adzukis are easier to digest than some other beans. This recipe is a new variation on the popular chili theme.

Makes one 5-ounce (150 gm) serving

½ cup (scant, 40%) adzuki beans
1 bay leaf
½ medium onion (120 gm) ½-inch diced
2 medium (12 gm.) garlic cloves—cut in half or as desired
½ teaspoon dried basil
1 teaspoon whole cumin seed
1 teaspoon (heaping) curry powder
3 ounces frozen mixed mushrooms
½ large red bell pepper, ½-inch diced
½ large green bell pepper, ½-inch diced
4 ounces canned whole Tuscan tomatoes, chopped (114 gm)

1. Steps 1 and 2 of Basic Beans Marinade (page 195), using adzuki beans and substituting 1 teaspoon of curry powder for the cardamom seed

2. Step 3 of Basic Beans Marinade.

3. Step 1 of Basic Beans Cooking (page 196), including *all* of the following: add the bay leaf, onion, garlic, basil, cumin seed, curry powder, and beans: Bring to a boil in a large pot.

4. Add the mushrooms and return to a boil.

5. Cover the pot and cook on low heat for five minutes or until beans are tender.

6. Add the tomatoes, stir until warm.

7. Remove bay leaf before serving.

LIGHT LENTILS

Lentils are the other exception to the overnight marination rule and should not be soaked before cooking. Lentils also yield a bit more cooked beans than other dried beans: 1 cup dried lentils → 2¼ cups cooked, 1 cup cooked lentils = 175 grams. Use about 3 cups water per 1 cup lentils.

Adzuki Chili	
Calories:	227.97
Protein (g):	11.37
Carbohydrates (g):	46.38
Sugars (g):	10.91
Glucose (g):	1.53
Fructose (g):	1.26
Dietary Fiber (g):	11.50
Fat (g):	0.86
Saturated Fat (g):	0.13
Phytosterols (mg):	16.11
Vit-A (mcg_RAE):	238.64
Carotene, beta (mcg):	1044.74
Carotene, alpha (mcg):	37.25
Cryptoxanthin, beta (mcg):	850.32
Lutein+zeaxanthin (mcg):	414.74
Vit-B1 Thiamine (mg):	0.21
Vit-B2 Riboflavin (mg):	0.11
Vit-B3 Niacin (mg):	1.39
Vit-B5 Pantothenic Acid (mg):	0.57
Vit-B6 Pyridoxine (mg):	0.46
Total Folate (mcg):	144.16
Vit-C (mg):	135.02
Tocopherol, Alpha (mg):	1.35
Vit-K (mcg):	14.58
Calcium (mg):	98.26
Magnesium (mg):	75.76
Phosphorus (mg):	216.63
Potassium (mg):	818.26
Sodium (mg):	149.15
Copper (mg):	0.43
Iron (mg):	4.11
Manganese (mg):	0.93
Selenium (mcg):	2.75

Makes four 5-ounce + (150 gm) servings

1 large bay leaf

1 medium onion (240 gm),

    ½-inch diced

6 medium garlic cloves (36 gm), cut in

    half or as desired

2 teaspoons whole cumin seeds

1 pound lentils, sorted to remove any

    small stones, rinsed, and drained

1½ teaspoons ground ginger, or to

    taste

Dressing for individual servings

3 teaspoons lemon juice

1½ teaspoons organic extra virgin

    olive oil

1 teaspoon flaxseeds, whole or ground,

    or the amount you prefer for fiber

    intake

Light Lentils	
Calories:	190.18
Protein (g):	14.07
Carbohydrates (g):	33.92
Sugars (g):	4.08
Glucose (g):	0.62
Fructose (g):	0.37
Dietary Fiber (g):	12.31
Fat (g):	0.64
Phytosterols (mg):	5.40
Vit-B1 Thiamine (mg):	0.27
Vit-B2 Riboflavin (mg):	0.121
Vit-B3 Niacin (mg):	1.65
Vit-B6 Pyridoxine (mg):	1
Total Folate (mcg):	276.06
Vitamin C (mg):	4.43
Vitamin E (IU):	0.25
Calcium (mg):	38.72
Magnesium (mg):	57.80
Phosphorus (mg):	283.56
Potassium (mg):	611.32
Sodium (mg):	4.24
Copper (mg):	0.4
Iron (mg):	5.01
Selenium (mcg):	4.66
Zinc (mg):	1.99

1. Bring 2 quarts water and the bay leaf to a boil in a large pot.

2. Add the onion, garlic, and cumin seeds—return to a medium boil for 5 minutes.

3. Add the lentils, return to a medium boil for 5 to 10 minutes, stirring occasionally. Check the consistency of the lentils. They can become overcooked and mushy quickly.

4. Just before removing from the heat, add the ground ginger and stir. Season to taste with additional ginger and garlic.

5. Remove the bay leaf before serving.

6. Plate individual servings of a scant ½ to ⅔ cup (100 to 150 gm), amount to meet protein-intake plan.

7. Add the individual dressing, stir, and serve.

CURRIED LIMA BEANS

While kohlrabi is delightful in this dish, if it is hard to find, you can substitute the same amount of turnip.

Serving Suggestions

- Serve as soup.
- Drain and serve as vegetable dish.
- Serve with or over barley.
- Serve with or over sprouted-grain bread.

In all cases, dress with organic extra virgin olive oil and lemon juice.

Makes four 5-ounce + servings (150 gm) with some left for tease meals

1 large bay leaf

1 medium onion (240 gm), ½-inch diced

Curried Lima Beans	
Calories:	132.76
Protein (g):	7.12
Carbohydrates (g):	25.28
Sugars (g):	2.63
Glucose (g):	0.65
Dietary Fiber (g):	6.55
Fat (g):	0.85
Saturated Fat (g):	0.10
Phytosterols (mg):	5.78
Vit-A IU:	149.76
Vit-B1 Thiamine (mg):	0.12
Vit-B5 Pantothenic Acid (mg):	0.26
Vit-B6 Pyridoxine (mg):	0.28
Total Folate (mcg):	31.45
Vit-C (mg):	36.03
Calcium (mg):	57.04
Magnesium (mg):	47.98
Phosphorus (mg):	110.87
Potassium (mg):	551.61
Sodium (mg):	46.42
Iron (mg):	3.09
Selenium (mcg):	2.67

6 medium garlic cloves (36 gm), cut in half or prepared as desired

2 teaspoons whole mustard seeds

1 medium-large kohlrabi (180 gm), 3/4-inch diced

1 10-ounce package organic frozen baby lima beans

1/4 teaspoon garlic powder or granules, or to taste

1/2 teaspoon curry powder, or to taste

Dressing for individual servings

1 to 2 teaspoons (5 to 10 gm) organic extra virgin olive oil, amount to meet fat-intake plan

2 to 4 teaspoons (5 to 10gm) lemon juice, generally twice the amount of olive oil, or to taste

1. Combine 2 cups water, bay leaf, onion, fresh garlic, mustard seed, and kohlrabi in a saucepan. Bring to a boil on low heat, 5 to 6 minutes.

2. Add the frozen baby lima beans and boil gently for 5 minutes, or until tender.

3. Add the curry powder and ground garlic as desired. Stir and taste.

4. Remove the bay leaf before serving.

5. Add olive oil and lemon juice to each serving.

EGGS AND MUNGS

Eggs, beans, and tomatoes have complementary flavors.

This is a recipe that demonstrates the benefit of cooking larger amounts of food than you need for immediate use. Having prepared Must-Have Mung Beans (pages 197-198), you are all set to quickly prepare this very pleasing egg dish.

The olive oil and lemon juice are listed separately to increase the flexibility of measuring and customizing the amount of fat you add.

Makes an individual serving

1 medium egg (57 gm), hard boiled, sliced or diced

½ cup (very scant) or 7 tablespoons (100 gm) Must-Have Mung Beans

½ cup (rounded) Tuscan Tomatoes (124 gm)

1 teaspoon (rounded) (½ gm) dried oregano, or to taste

Shakes of garlic to taste

Dressing

¾ teaspoon (4 gm) olive oil, or the amount that matches your fat intake plans

1½ teaspoons lemon juice, or to taste

Eggs and Mungs	
Calories:	219.93
Protein (g)	15.11
Carbohydrates (g):	25.84
Sugars (g)	6.70
Dietary Fiber (g):	8.60
Fat (g):	6.07
Saturated Fat (g):	1.88
Monounsaturated Fat (g):	2.21
Polyunsaturated Fat (g):	0.91
Cholesterol (mg):	241.11
Vit-A (mcg. RAE):	125.00
Vit-B1 Thiamine (mg):	0.19
Vit-B2 Riboflavin (mg):	0.31
Vit-B5 Pantothenic Acid (mg):	1.05
Vit-B6 Pyridoxine (mg):	0.13
Total Folate (mcg):	178.95
Vit-B12 Cyanocobalamin (mcg):	0.46
Vit-C (mg):	22.00
Vit-E (IU):	1.65
Calcium (mg):	76.93
Magnesium (mg):	53.70
Phosphorus (mg):	199.89
Potassium (mg):	334.40
Sodium (mg):	161.60
Copper (mg):	0.16
Iron (mg):	2.35
Manganese (mg):	0.31
Selenium (mcg):	20.06
Zinc (mg):	1.47

1. Place all the ingredients in a bowl or ramekin. Stir.

2. Serve or place in a water bath until ready to serve.

LEMON-GINGER SALMON

Serving Suggestion

Lemon-Ginger Salmon served with barley is a family favorite.

Combine Lemon-Ginger Salmon with 1 to 1⅓ cups of Savory Barley (page 205), tailoring the serving size to the CR level you choose.

Makes an individual serving

2 to 2½ ounces wild-caught Alaskan salmon—fresh, poached, or canned (water-packed with bones and no added salt)

1½ tablespoons lemon juice

⅛ teaspoon ground ginger, or to taste

1 teaspoon EVO (5 gm), or amount to meet calorie and fat intake goals

1. If using **canned salmon,** mix all ingredients in an individual dish and enjoy.

   For poached salmon, put a cup of water (or mix with white wine) in a sauté pan.

2. Bring to a simmer on medium heat.

3 Place salmon fillets, skin-side down in the pan.

Lemon-Ginger Salmon	
Calories:	146.78
Protein (g):	14.10
Carbohydrates (g):	2.26
Sugars (g):	0.54
Dietary Fiber (g):	0.29
Fat (g):	9.02
Saturated Fat (g):	1.76
Monounsaturated Fat (g):	4.96
Polyunsaturated Fat (g):	1.80
Omega-3 (g):	1.22
Omega-6 (g):	0.11
Vit-A (mcg_RAE):	12.27
Vit-A IU:	43.53
Vit-B3 Niacin (mg):	4.67
Vit-B5 Pantothenic Acid (mg):	0.41
Vit-B6 Pyridoxine (mg):	0.22
Total Folate (mcg):	12.88
Vit-B12 Cyanocobalamin (mcg):	3.12
Vit-C (mg):	5.58
Tocopherol, Alpha (mg):	0.03
Calcium (mg):	154.15
Magnesium (mg):	25.88
Phosphorus (mg):	235.07
Potassium (mg):	268.87
Sodium (mg):	58.05
Iron (mg):	0.82
Manganese (mg):	0.02
Selenium (mcg):	23.54
Zinc (mg):	0.67

4. Cook 5 minutes or to desired done-ness. Do not overcook.

5. Dress the salmon with the other ingredients. Enjoy as is or add Savory Barley and mix.

GRAINS

SAVORY BARLEY

Barley is versatile, nutritious and extremely low in glycemic effect. It is particularly delicious both as a savory carbohydrate itself and as an ingredient in savory veggie dishes. A fact that is not always easy to find is the equivalents between dry measures of grain and the cooked yield. So: 1 cup dried barley→2 to 3 cups cooked. A good rule of thumb is to use about 4 cups water per cup of barley.

Overnight marination of the barley and spices blends the flavors and shortens cooking time, thus reducing production of AGE (Advanced Glycation Endproducts, on page 68, Chapter 4: "Glucose Control").

Makes four 5-ounce + (150-gm) servings

For the Marinade
  1 bay leaf
  1 pound of dried hulled barley (or hull-less, see Glossary and "Foods to Choose" chapter)
  2 teaspoons whole cardamom seeds
  2 teaspoons whole cumin seeds
  2 teaspoons whole yellow mustard seeds

For cooking
  1 bay leaf
  1 medium onion (240 gm), sliced or ½-inch diced

6 medium (36 gm) garlic cloves—cut in half, or as desired

2 portabella mushroom caps (140 grams), sliced

2 teaspoons whole or ground cardamom seeds

2 teaspoons whole or ground cumin seeds

2 teaspoons whole or ground mustard seeds

Marinade

Mix all marinade ingredients in a bowl and add enough water to cover one-half inch over the grain. Marinate it in the refrigerator overnight.

Cooking

1. Drain the grain in a colander.

2. Place all the the Savory Barley cooking ingredients *except* the mushrooms in a large pot with enough water to cover 1/2 inch over the grain.

3. Bring to a boil uncovered. Boil gently for 6 minutes.

4. Add the mushrooms. Bring back to a boil, stirring the grain from the bottom to give all the barley access to heat and water. Boil gently, uncovered, for 4 minutes.

Savory Barley	
Calories:	129.60
Protein (g):	3.06
Carbohydrates (g):	28.86
Sugars (g):	4.26
Glucose (g):	0.26
Fructose (g):	0.16
Dietary Fiber (g):	6.16
Fat (g):	0.28
Saturated Fat (g):	0.06
Monounsaturated Fat (g):	0.04
Polyunsaturated Fat (g):	0.14
Omega-3 (g):	0.01
Omega-6 (g):	0.12
Phytosterols (mg):	2.03
Carotene, beta (mcg):	2.92
Lutein+zeaxanthin (mcg):	33.06
Vit-B1 Thiamine (mg):	1.34
Vit-B2 Riboflavin (mg):	1.28
Vit-B3 Niacin (mg):	1.31
Vit-B5 Pantothenic Acid (mg):	0.12
Vit-B6 Pyridoxine (mg):	0.14
Total Folate (mcg):	11.62
Vit-C (mg):	2.25
Calcium (mg):	26.56
Magnesium (mg):	14.73
Phosphorus (mg):	40.54
Potassium (mg):	117.42
Sodium (mg):	6.10
Iron (mg):	1.44
Manganese (mg):	0.24
Selenium (mcg):	5.49

5. Reduce the heat to low and cover.

6. Simmer, covered, for 5 to 10 minutes, stirring occasionally, adding water as needed to keep barley covered.

7. Taste the grain and use ground cardamom, cumin, and mustard seeds to adjust the flavor.

8. Simmer, covered, for another 5 to 10 minutes, stirring occasionally.

9. Test the grain for doneness. Continue to simmer till the grain is tender.

10. Set off the heat until the water is absorbed. Stir occasionally.

11. It will be ready to eat in 20 minutes.

12. Remove the bay leaf before serving.

SAVORY BARLEY-VEGGIE COMBO

Serving Suggestion

- Combine serving of Savory Barley—7½ to 10 ounces (200 to 300 gm), depending on the level of calorie restriction you choose, in a bowl with 5¼ to 7½ (adjust to your preferences) of frozen vegetables such as broccoli, green beans, or a vegetable mix—in proportion to the barley.
- Add dressing ingredients and place bowl in a water bath until ready to serve.

Substitution

If you prefer to replace frozen veggies with fresh, increase cooking time accordingly.

Makes four servings

1 large bay leaf

1 medium onion (240 gm), 1/2-inch diced

6 medium garlic cloves (36 gm)—cut in half or prepared as desired

1 package (7 1/2 ounces) frozen broccoli

1 package (10-ounce) frozen bell peppers—red, yellow, and green

2 1/2 to 3 3/4 cups Savory Barley (200 to 300 gm)

Garlic powder or granules to taste

Dressing for individual servings

1 1/2 to 3 1/2 ounces low-sodium, organic vegetable cocktail (Knudsen's Very Veggie), or stewed tomatoes (no salt added), fresh or canned, depending on your taste preference

1/2 teaspoon crushed oregano leaves, or to taste

1 1/2 teaspoons organic extra virgin olive oil

1 tablespoon + 1/2 teaspoon lemon juice, or to taste

Garlic powder or granules to taste

2 1/2 to 3 3/4 cups Savory Barley (200 to 300 gm)

1. Bring a quart of water with the bay leaf to a boil in a large pot.

2. Add the onion and garlic— return to a medium boil for 5 minutes.

Savory Barley Veggie Combo	
Calories:	307.86
Protein (g):	7.14
Carbohydrates (g):	69.73
Sugars (g):	5.47
Glucose (g):	1.47
Fructose (g):	0.70
Dietary Fiber (g):	10.40
Fat (g):	0.97
Phytosterols (mg):	9.0
Vit-A (mcg. RAE):	12.53
Lutein + zeaxanthin (mcg):	117.34
Vit-B1 Thiamine (mg):	0.21
Vit-B2 Riboflavin (mg):	0.15
Vit-B3 Niacin (mg):	4.24
Vit-B5 Pantothenic Acid (mg):	0.40
Vit-B6 Pyridoxine (mg):	0.43
Total Folate (mcg):	43.67
Vit-C (mg):	64.77
Vit-K (mcg):	1.97
Calcium (mg):	68.99
Magnesium (mg):	52.25
Phosphorus (mg):	137.97
Potassium (mg):	308.62
Sodium (mg):	21.83
Copper (mg):	0.26
Iron (mg):	3.18
Manganese (mg):	0.57
Selenium (mcg):	18.78
Zinc (mg):	1.84

3. Add the vegetables—return to medium boil for 3 minutes.

4. Add the bell peppers; return to the beginnings of the boil for 3 minutes; the vegetables will be tender.

5. Remove the bay leaf before serving. Drain. Reserve the broth for later use.

6. Serve over barley with garnishes listed above

SWEET WHEAT BERRIES

Wheat berries are not actually sweet, but they do complement sweeter foods—fruit, for example—very naturally. So, one of the places you'll find them here is in the dessert recipes. They also accompany both sweet potatoes and beets very well.

Makes 3 servings of almost 4½ ounces (125 gm) with some left for tease meals

For the marinade

   1 pound dried wheat berries
   2 teaspoons pumpkin pie spice (cinnamon, ginger, cloves, and nutmeg—combined)

For the cooking

   2 teaspoons pumpkin pie spice

Marinade

1. Rinse the wheat berries in a colander until the water is clear.

2. Place the wheat berries in a large bowl, adding pumpkin pie spice and water to cover the grain by 1/2 inch. Stir.

3. Marinate overnight in the refrigerator.

Cooking

1. Drain.

2. Bring 8 cups water to a boil in a pot.

3. Add the wheat berries; return to a boil, reduce the heat to low.

4. Cover and cook for 20 to 30 minutes, or until tender.

5. Add 2 more teaspoons pumpkin pie spice and mix.

6. Serve warm. Cool the rest and put into containers for refrigeration or freezing.

After cooking, let stand covered for delicious extra plumping of the wheat berries as they absorb the remaining water.

Sweet Wheat Berries	
Calories:	186.76
Protein (g):	5.49
Carbohydrates (g):	40.71
Dietary Fiber (g):	2.85
Fat (g):	
Saturated Fat (g):	0.49
Phytosterols (mg):	4.83
Vit-B1 Thiamine (mg):	0.53
Vit-B2 Riboflavin (mg):	0.20
Vit-B3 Niacin (mg):	8.55
Vit-B5 Pantothenic Acid (mg):	1.65
Vit-B6 Pyridoxine (mg):	0.55
Total Folate (mcg):	34.97
Tocopherol, Alpha (mg):	2.16
Vit-K (mcg):	46.93
Calcium (mg):	59.28
Phosphorus (mg):	143.47
Potassium (mg):	108.98
Sodium (mg):	4.38
Chromium (mcg):	0.60
Copper (mg):	0.18
Iodine (mcg):	1.35
Iron (mg):	3.08
Manganese (mg):	2.88
Selenium (mcg):	2.67
Zinc (mg):	1.56

WHEAT BERRY CEREAL

This recipe is an *individual serving* to match what you would normally do to prepare cereal.

½ cup (scant) (100 gm) Sweet Wheat Berries, page 209

½ cup (scant) fruit, e.g., frozen organic blueberries, raspberries, strawberries, blackberries, in any combination (100 gm)

⅔ teaspoon olive oil (3 gm)

2 to 3 walnut halves (5 gm)

2 to 3 teaspoons lemon juice (10 to 15 gm), or to taste

1. Place the wheat berries in an individual bowl.

2. Water-bathe the berries, if you prefer to serve them warm.

3. Add the remaining ingredients.

4. Stir and serve.

Wheat Berry Cereal	
Calories:	268.72
Protein (g):	6.56
Carbohydrates (g):	49.74
Sugars (g):	4.50
Dietary Fiber (g):	6.83
Fat (g):	6.40
Saturated Fat (g):	0.71
Monounsaturated Fat (g):	1.06
Polyunsaturated Fat (g):	1.48
Vit-B1 Thiamine (mg):	0.52
Vit-B2 Riboflavin (mg):	0.19
Vit-B3 Niacin (mg):	8.40
Vit-B5 Pantothenic Acid (mg):	1.65
Vit-B6 Pyridoxine (mg):	0.52
Total Folate (mcg):	31.50
Vit-C (mg):	15.75
Tocopherol, Alpha (mg):	2.10
Vit-K (mcg):	45.00
Calcium (mg):	32.35
Magnesium (mg):	5.65
Phosphorus (mg):	229.52
Potassium (mg):	143.45
Sodium (mg):	1.34
Chromium (mcg):	0.60
Copper (mg):	0.22
Iodine (mcg):	1.35
Iron (mg):	2.40
Manganese (mg):	1.91
Selenium (mcg):	2.04
Zinc (mg):	1.54

SOUPS

BARLEY SOUP

The most common barley soup is made with mushrooms. But that's just the beginning. Following are several varieties of barley soup that are quite distinct from each other.

FLORAL-FLAVORED BARLEY SOUP

This recipe is designed to be served over Savory Barley (pages 205–206).

The wonderful floral flavor of this soup is due to celery root— which is also known as celeriac or celery knob. It is somewhat less than beautiful to the eye, but when it is lightly cooked, it gives a distinctive flavor. Some say it's a cross between parsley and celery, two of its relatives. Because of its floral aroma and flavor, it complements vegetables like bell peppers very well.

The cardamom, lemon grass, and tarragon add to the aromatic delight.

If whole, dried cardamom seed is unavailable, substitute 2 teaspoons of ground cardamom.

Makes six 5-ounce + (150 gm) servings

- 2 teaspoons whole dried cardamom seeds
- 2 teaspoons dried tarragon
- 1 teaspoon dried lemon grass
- 1 medium onion (240 gm), ½-inch diced
- 1 medium celery root (250 gm), ⅓-inch diced

Floral-Flavored Barley Soup	
Calories:	184.00
Protein (g):	5.27
Carbohydrates (g):	33.05
Sugars (g):	10.89
Glucose (g):	2.58
Fructose (g):	1.53
Dietary Fiber (g):	6.64
Fat (g):	4.47
Saturated Fat (g):	0.42
Monounsaturated Fat (g):	0.58
Polyunsaturated Fat (g):	2.96
Omega-3 (g):	0.55
Omega-6 (g):	2.41
Phytosterols (mg):	26.60
Vit-A (mcg. RAE):	25.00
Lutein + zeaxanthin (mcg):	15.82
Vit-B1 Thiamine (mg):	0.55
Vit-B2 Riboflavin (mg):	0.51
Vit-B3 Niacin (mg):	1.29
Vit-B5 Pantothenic Acid (mg):	0.46
Vit-B6 Pyridoxine (mg):	0.36
Total Folate (mcg):	31.51
Vit-C (mg):	82.82
Tocopherol, Gamma (mg):	1.25
Tocopherol, Delta (mg):	0.11
Calcium (mg):	83.64
Magnesium (mg):	42.59
Phosphorus (mg):	158.77
Potassium (mg):	481.06
Sodium (mg):	82
Copper (mg):	0.25
Iron (mg):	1.54
Manganese (mg):	0.59
Selenium (mcg):	3.33

1 10-ounce package frozen bell peppers, yellow, red, and green, mixed

½ cup (scant) (100 gm) Savory Barley per serving, or more to match your chosen percentage of CR

Garnish

5 to 6 walnut halves per serving (12 gm)

1½ tablespoons lime juice

1. Bring 2 quarts water with cardamom seeds, tarragon, lemon grass, and onion to a boil.

2. Boil gently, uncovered for 5 minutes, or until the pungency of the onion aroma reduces.

3. Add the celery root. Continue to boil on medium heat for 5 minutes, or until the celery root is tender.

4. Add the bell peppers. Bring back to the very beginning of the boil.

5. Pour over the barley and serve with walnuts.

TOMATO-VEGGIE BARLEY SOUP

This soup can be served warm or cool, depending on the season and your preference. To heat, use a water bath to gently warm the soup. This recipe is presented by the *individual serving* because it is composed of all ready-to-use or pre-prepared food. Tuscan Tomatoes are listed because they contain very little sodium.

Makes 8 servings with some left for tease meals

⅔ to 1 cup (150 to 200 gm) low
glycemic vegetables, according to
your preference

Vegetable broth, your preferred amount

½ cup (scant) (100 gm) whole canned
tomatoes

½ cup (scant) (100 gm) Savory Barley

⅔ to 1 cup (150 to 227 gm) Very
Veggie (Knudsen's) low-sodium,
organic vegetable cocktail,
depending on use of broth and your
preference for degree of soupiness

½ teaspoon oregano, or to taste

1 to 2 teaspoons (5 to 10 gm) extra virgin olive oil (EVO), depending on taste
and intended fat intake

2 to 4 teaspoons (1 tablespoon + 1 teaspoon) (2 times the amount of EVO)
lemon juice

Tomato-Veggie Barley Soup	
Calories:	259.53
Protein (g):	7.04
Carbohydrates (g):	44.01
Sugars (g):	14.65
Glucose (g):	0.28
Fructose (g):	0.19
Dietary Fiber (g):	11.27
Fat (g):	5.20
Saturated Fat (g):	0.77
Monosaturated fat (g):	3.37
Polyunsaturated fat (g):	1.35
Vit-A (mcg_RAE):	254.79
Carotene, beta (mcg):	2500
Carotene, alpha (mcg):	1125
Lycopene (mcg):	0.60
Lutein + zeaxanthin (mcg):	262.54
Vit-B1 Thiamine (mg):	1
Vit-B2 Riboflavin (mg):	0.93
Vit-B3 Niacin (mg):	2.16
Total Folate (mcg):	34.95
Vit-C (mg):	64.43
Tocopherol, Alpha (mg):	0.43
Vit-K (mcg):	12.91
Calcium (mg):	90.27
Magnesium (mg):	35.49
Phosphorus (mg):	54.74
Potassium (mg):	1145.17
Sodium (mg):	84.13
Copper (mg):	0.10
Iron (mg):	3.37
Manganese (mg):	0.36
Selenium (mcg):	4.21

1. Mix the first five ingredients in an individual bowl.

2. Add the next three ingredients directly or taste them as you
   go until you achieve your preferred proportions.

3. Serve or put in a water bath if serving warm.

PEA SOUP WITH TARRAGON

Serving Suggestions

- Serve immediately as soup or drain and serve as vegetable dish.
- If you are not using all the soup at the moment, drain remaining vegetables, reserving the broth. Save vegetables and broth separately to use as soup, as vegetable dish, or as ingredients.

Makes four 5-ounce+ (150 gm) servings with some left for tease meals

Pea Soup with Tarragon	
Calories:	88.23
Protein (g):	4.27
Carbohydrates (g):	18.29
Sugars (g):	4.97
Glucose (g):	1.08
Fructose (g):	0.64
Dietary Fiber (g):	4.86
Fat (g):	0.09
Phytosterols (mg):	8.30
Vit-A (IU):	359.24
Vit-B5 Pantothenic Acid (mg):	0.78
Vit-C (mg):	8.73
Calcium (mg):	36
Magnesium (mg):	5.57
Phosphorus (mg):	15.26
Potassium (mg):	113.69
Sodium (mg):	166.46
Copper (mg):	0.21
Iron (mg):	1.13
Selenium (mcg):	5.17

1 large bay leaf

1 medium-large onion (240 gm)

2 teaspoon ground dried tarragon

2 teaspoons dried basil

1½ teaspoons ground dried rosemary or 2½ teaspoons fresh rosemary, chopped

10 ounces fresh shiitake mushrooms or 1 10-ounce package frozen shiitake mushrooms

1 pound fresh or frozen organic peas

1. Add the bay leaf, onion, tarragon, basil, and rosemary to a saucepan with 6 to 8 cups water. Bring water to a boil. Boil for 3 minutes.

2. Add the mushrooms. Return to a boil. Boil for 3 minutes on medium heat.

3. Add the peas. Return to a boil. Boil lightly for 1 to 3 minutes or until tender.

4. Remove the bay leaf before serving.

CARDAMOM-FLAVORED VEGETABLE SOUP

This particularly heartwarming soup can be served over Savory Barley or spouted-grain bread. It can also be drained and served as a vegetable dish. Bok choy has a nice crunch and is high in calcium, but if it's not available, other greens add their own distinctive flavors, e.g., collard greens, kale, Swiss chard. When cleaning these greens, removing the fibrous "veins" will give you less gratuitous fiber, making the greens easier to digest. The peppers will cook a bit faster, so add them a few minutes after the other vegetables.

Makes four 5-ounce + (150 gm) servings

1 bay leaf
3 medium garlic cloves (18 gm)

Cardamom-Flavored Vegetable Soup	
Calories:	77.86
Protein (g):	4.23
Carbohydrates (g):	16.01
Sugars (g):	7.35
Glucose (g):	1.14
Fructose (g):	.70
Dietary Fiber (g):	6.35
Fat (g):	0.48
Phytosterols:	8.64
Vit-A (mcg RAE):	202.32
Carotene, beta (mcg):	1911.66
Carotene, alpha (mcg):	1040.40
Lycopene (mcg):	0.72
Lutein + zeaxanthin (mcg):	122.44
Total Folate:	40.27
Vit-C (mg):	87.45
Tocopherol, alpha (mg):	0.50
Vit-K (mcg):	12.91
Calcium (mg):	66.56
Phosphorus (mg):	51.18
Potassium (mg):	303.89
Sodium (mg):	52.16
Iron (mg):	1.10
Molybdenum (mcg):	22.40
Selenium (mcg):	1.27

1 tablespoon + 1 teaspoon whole cardamom seeds

2 teaspoons dried or fresh (well rinsed) rosemary

2 teaspoons dried marjoram

1 cup bok choy (Chinese cabbage) (250 gm)

2 1-pound packages frozen low glycemic vegetables, or 2 pounds fresh mixed carrots, broccoli, cauliflower, green beans

10 ounces fresh bell peppers, or 1 10-ounce package bell peppers, red, yellow, and green

1. Add the bay leaf, garlic, cardamom seeds, rosemary, marjoram, and 10 cups water to a pot.

2. Bring to a boil. Boil on medium heat for 5 minutes.

3. Add the bok choy. Cook on medium heat for 2 minutes.

4. Add the mixed vegetables and peppers. Bring back to a boil.

5. If the vegetables were frozen, they are ready to be served. If fresh, boil them over medium heat until just tender to a fork.

POTLUCK VEGETABLE SOUP

Especially since this is "potluck," you have many options. Here are a few: If kohlrabi is not available, add a vegetable with low or medium Glycemic Index ranking, e.g.:

Turnip 1 medium (120 gm), 1/2-inch diced

Black radish 1 small to medium (120 to 150 gm), 1/2-inch diced

Red radishes 1/4 to 1/3 pound (120 to 180 gm), 1/2-inch diced

If celery root is not available, add two large bell peppers of different colors if available, 3/4-inch diced.

Makes ten 5-ounce+ (150 gm), servings providing the opportunity to refrigerate and freeze some for later use or to serve friends

- 1 large bay leaf
- 2 teaspoons mustard seeds
- 1 tablespoon cardamom seeds
- 1 large onion (360 gm), ½-inch diced
- 12 garlic cloves (72 gm), cut in half or size as desired
- 1 medium or medium-large kohlrabi (120 to 180 gm), peeled to remove all green and ½-inch diced
- 1 large celery root (800 gm), ½-inch diced
- 1 16-ounce package frozen mixed low glycemic vegetables, e.g., carrots, broccoli, cauliflower, green beans, bell peppers, or fresh if local

Pot Luck Vegetable Soup	
Calories:	29.47
Protein (g):	1.0
Carbohydrates (g):	6.23
Sugars (g):	1.71
Glucose (g):	0.46
Fructose (g):	0.27
Dietary Fiber (g):	1.62
Fat (g):	0.27
Phytosterols (mg):	4.10
Vit-A (mcg_RAE):	14.71
Carotene, beta (mcg):	144.85
Carotene, alpha (mcg):	63.64
Lutein + zeaxanthin (mcg):	18.47
Vit-B1 Thiamine (mg):	0.15
Vit-B2 Riboflavin (mg):	0.14
Vit-C (mg):	13.97
Vit-K (mcg):	4.73
Calcium (mg):	24.87
Magnesium (mg):	10.23
Phosphorus (mg):	35.22
Potassium (mg):	138.62
Sodium (mg):	15.76
Selenium (mcg):	1.61

Dressing for individual servings

- 1 tablespoon organic extra virgin olive oil
- 2 tablespoons lemon juice

1. In a large soup pot, bring 6 to 8 cups water to a boil, add bay leaf, mustard and cardamom seeds, onion, garlic, kohlrabi, and celery root and boil moderately for 5 minutes, or until the kohlrabi is just starting to be tender.

2. Add the mixed vegetables and cook until they simmer.

3. Dress and serve if the vegetables were frozen, removing the bay leaf before serving.

3a. Boil on low heat until tender if the vegetables were fresh. Dress and serve, removing the bay leaf before serving.

MUSHROOM MAGIC CANCER-FIGHTING SOUP

Both maitake and shiitake mushrooms are widely available in health food stores.

Serving Suggestions

- Serve as soup.
- Serve soup over sprouted-grain bread or Savory Barley.

Makes five 5-ounce+ (150 gm) servings with some left for tease meals

1 medium onion (240 gm), ½-inch diced

6 medium garlic cloves (36 gm), cut in half or prepared as desired

2 medium-large kohlrabi (300 gm), cleaned, peeled, and cut into ¾-inch pieces

2 medium turnips (200 to 300 gm), cleaned and cut into ¾-inch pieces

2 maitake mushrooms, (8 ounces), rinsed, ¾-inch pieces

Mushroom Magic Cancer-Fighting Soup	
Calories:	70.06
Protein (g):	3.14
Carbohydrates (g):	15.81
Sugars (g):	4.11
Glucose (g):	0.40
Fructose (g):	0.24
Dietary Fiber (g):	5.79
Fat (g):	0.17
Phytosterols (mg):	6.28
Vit-B1 Thiamine (mg):	0.11
Vit-B2 Riboflavin (mg):	0.11
Vit-B3 Niacin (mg):	3.16
Vit-B5 Pantothenic Acid (mg):	0.81
Vit-B6 Pyridoxine (mg):	0.20
Total Folate (mcg):	19.85
Vit-C (mg):	46.77
Vit-D (IU):	78.61
Tocopherol, Alpha (mg):	0.29
Calcium (mg):	37.80
Magnesium (mg):	23.08
Phosphorus (mg):	82.56
Potassium (mg):	474.57
Sodium (mg):	43.58
Copper (mg):	0.28
Iron (mg):	0.66
Selenium (mcg):	5.24

1 10-ounce package frozen shiitake mushrooms, or 10 ounces fresh shiitake mushrooms

Garnish for individual servings

1 teaspoon organic extra virgin olive oil (5 gm)

2 teaspoons lemon juice (10 gm)

1. In a large pot bring 2 to 3 cups water to a boil.

2. Add the onion, garlic, and kohlrabi. Boil gently, 5 to 6 minutes.

3. Add the turnip and mushrooms. Boil gently, 4 minutes.

4. If not to be used immediately, drain the vegetables, reserving the broth. Store separately. This stops the cooking and increases flexibility of use.

Mushroom Magic Soup with Garnish	
Calories:	111.34
Protein (g):	3.19
Carbohydrates (g):	16.10
Sugars (g):	4.19
Glucose (g):	0.41
Fructose (g):	0.24
Dietary Fiber (g):	5.89
Fat (g):	4.85
Saturated Fat (g):	0.69
Monounsaturated Fat (g):	3.34
Polyunsaturated Fat (g):	0.74
Phytosterols (mg):	6.40
Vit-B1 Thiamine (mg):	0.12
Vit-B2 Riboflavin (mg):	0.11
Vit-B3 Niacin (mg):	3.22
Vit-B5 Pantothenic Acid (mg):	0.82
Vit-B6 Pyridoxine (mg):	0.20
Total Folate (mcg):	20.21
Vit-C (mg):	47.63
Vit-D (IU):	80.05
Tocopherol, Alpha (mg):	0.29
Vit-K (mcg):	0.24
Calcium (mg):	38.49
Magnesium (mg):	23.51
Phosphorus (mg):	84.07
Potassium (mg):	483.25
Sodium (mg):	44.38
Copper (mg):	0.28
Iron (mg):	0.67
Manganese (mg):	0.23
Selenium (mcg):	5.34

CARDAMOM-FLAVORED VEGETABLE SOUP

This is a family favorite.

Makes four 5-ounce+ (150 gm) servings

- 1 medium onion (240 gm)
- 6 medium garlic cloves (36 gm), cut in half or as preferred
- 4 teaspoons (19 gm) whole cardamom seeds
- 2 teaspoons dried rosemary, ground in a seed or coffee grinder
- 2 teaspoons dried marjoram
- 1 cup (250 gm) bok choy, cut or broken into bite size pieces
- 2 16-ounce packages frozen mixed (low GI) vegetables, or fresh vegetables if local
- 10 ounces frozen bell peppers, preferably mixed colors, or fresh if local

Dressing for individual servings

- 1 tablespoon organic extra virgin olive oil
- 2 tablespoons lemon juice

1. Add the onion, garlic, cardamom seeds, rosemary, and marjoram to 10 cups water (2½ quarts) in a pot.

2. Bring to a boil. Boil over low heat for 5 minutes.

Cardamom-Flavored Vegetable Soup	
Calories:	79.80
Protein (g):	2.39
Carbohydrates (g):	0.14
Sugars (g):	2.29
Glucose (g):	0.08
Fructose (g):	0.06
Dietary Fiber (g):	4.52
Fat (g):	3.85
Saturated Fat (g):	0.58
Vit: A (mcg_RAE):	189.93
Carotene, beta (mcg):	1853.20
Carotene, alpha (mcg):	834.56
Lycopene (mcg):	0.44
Lutein+zeaxanthin (mcg):	179.56
Vit-B1 Thiamine (mg):	0.43
Vit-B2 Riboflavin (mg):	0.44
Vit-C (mg):	36.86
Vit- K (mcg):	9.36
Calcium (mg):	68.64
Phosphorus (mg):	27.74
Potassium (mg):	144.48
Sodium (mg):	44.27
Iron (mg):	1.19
Selenium (mcg):	1.06

3. Add the bok choy. Cook on medium heat for 2 minutes.

4. Add the vegetables and peppers.

5. Bring back to a boil.

6. Serve if the vegetables were frozen.
   Boil on low heat until tender if the vegetables were fresh.

7. Remove the bay leaf before serving.

8. Dress and serve.

SIMPLE VEGETABLE SOUP

This soup is delightful and easy. The hardest thing is peeling four garlic cloves and peeling and cutting up the turnip. But leave the clean, purple skin on the turnip to get those phytonutrients. Fines herbes is a classic French seasoning blend of chervil, chives, parsley, and tarragon that adds a gardeny freshness, especially to fish and vegetables. This soup is great on its own or served over Savory Barley or sprouted-grain bread. It is also a very nice vegetable dish if strained, reserving the broth. The barley and bread are then good optional accompaniments.

The dressing enhances the flavors and the nutritional balance.

Simple Vegetable Soup	
Calories:	50.91
Protein (g):	2.40
Carbohydrates (g):	10.48
Sugars (g):	4.87
Glucose (g):	0.32
Fructose (g):	0.19
Dietary Fiber (g):	3.14
Fat (g):	0.04
Saturated Fat (g)	0.01
Phytosterols (mg):	4.22
Vit-A IU:	96.39
Vit-C (mg):	26.33
Calcium (mg):	32.39
Phosphorus (mg):	12.92
Potassium (mg):	76.40
Sodium (mg):	28.14
Iron (mg):	0.47
Selenium (mcg):	0.41

Makes eleven 5-ounce+ (150 gm) servings

1 medium onion (240 gm)

2 teaspoons fines herbes

4 garlic cloves (24 gm)

10 ounces organic mushrooms or 1 10-ounce package frozen organic mixed mushrooms

10 ounces (285 gm) organic turnip

1 pound organic broccoli florets or 1 16-ounce package frozen

1 pound organic green beans or 1 16-ounce package frozen

Dressing for individual servings

1 teaspoon (5 gm) organic extra virgin olive oil, or your choice, depending on
   your fat-intake goal

2 teaspoons (10 gm) lemon juice, or 2 times the amount of olive oil you choose

1. Add the onion, fines herbes, garlic, mushrooms, and 4 cups (1 quart) water to a pot.

2. Bring to a boil. Boil on medium heat for 3 minutes.

3. Add the turnip. Bring back to a boil.

4. Add the fresh vegetables and bring back to a boil. Boil on medium heat until tender. If using frozen vegetables, cook over medium heat until they start to simmer.

5. If you will have some soup left over, drain the vegetables to stop the cooking and store them separately from the broth. Both can be used later, separately or together.

SWEET PEPPER AND CABBAGE SOUP

This soup is complemented by the sprouted-grain bread. If you make more soup than will be used immediately, draining and refrigerating the vegetables separately from the broth stops the cooking, leaving the veggies more al dente. Later, the broth and vegetables can be used separately or together as soup.

Makes eight 5-ounce+ (150 gm) servings

1 large bay leaf
2 teaspoons whole cardamom seeds
1 medium onion (240 gm)
1/2 small head cabbage (1 pound)
1 medium celery root (250 gm)
10 ounces bell peppers, mixed colors, fresh or frozen
3 broken walnut halves (6 gm)

1. Bring the bay leaf, cardamom seeds, onion, cabbage, and celery root to a boil in 1 1/2 quarts of water. Boil for 5 minutes on medium heat.

2. Add the peppers. Bring back to a boil and boil for 2 minutes on medium heat.

3. Add the walnuts and mix just before serving.

4. Dish and serve.

Sweet Pepper and Cabbage Soup	
Calories:	45.18
Protein (g):	1.73
Carbohydrates (g):	9.05
Sugars (g):	3.06
Dietary Fiber (g):	2.68
Fat (g):	0.78
Phytosterols (mg):	11.64
Vit-A IU:	557.60
Vit-B5 Pantothenic Acid (mg):	0.20
Vit-B6 Pyridoxine (mg):	0.20
Total Folate (mcg):	46.80
Vit-C (mg):	87.93
Calcium (mg):	44.18
Magnesium (mg):	19.83
Phosphorus (mg):	52.24
Potassium (mg):	303.78
Sodium (mg):	31.28
Chromium (mcg):	0.18
Iodine (mcg):	0.12
Manganese (mg):	0.22
Molybdenum (mcg):	8.48
Selenium (mcg):	0.92

THE CR WAY SANDWICHES

The CR Way Sandwiches are delectable open-faced pleasures that we treat ourselves to almost every day. Their flexibility will allow you to use them to meet your nutrient goals as well as your enjoyment quota. The base of every *The CR Way* Sandwich is the Essential Sandwich.

ESSENTIAL SANDWICH

Several variations on the *The CR Way* Sandwich theme can be found on the pages that follow. Each sandwich variation makes an individual serving, which can easily be doubled, tripled, etc., as desired. If you prefer deep-dish sandwiches, use the same ingredients and amounts as for the individual sandwiches. Put all the ingredients into a dish, ramekin, or jar, pour lemon juice and olive oil, stir to distribute. This reduces preparation time and facilitates packing food for travel.

1 slice sprouted-grain bread (31 to 41 gm)

1 tablespoon lemon juice (14 gm)

1 to 2 tablespoons vegetable broth, as needed to further moisten bread

1½ teaspoons organic extra virgin olive oil (7 gm)

Optional: 2-3 walnut halves (depending on how much fat you are including in your CR plan)

1 teaspoon flaxseeds, whole or ground (depending on how much fiber you are including in your CR plan)

Your favorite herbs and spices, depending on the topping

Essential Sandwich	
Calories:	90.02
Protein (g):	3.00
Carbohydrates (g):	3.75
Dietary Fiber (g):	8.25
Fat (g):	5.00
Saturated Fat (g):	0.50
Monounsaturated Fat (g):	2.50
Polyunsaturated Fat (g):	0.50
Vit-B2 Riboflavin (mg):	0.53
Vit-B3 Niacin (mg):	0.90
Total Folate (mcg):	9.60
Magnesium (mg):	26.26
Phosphorus (mg):	43.51
Potassium (mg):	75.02
Sodium (mg):	48.76
Iron (mg):	0.27
Zinc (mg):	0.28

Since the walnut halves are optional, the nutrient boxes do not include nutrients from them.

1. Place the slice of bread on a plate.

2. Drizzle the lemon juice over the bread. Use reserved vegetable broth if the crust is hard and needs more moistening.

3. Drizzle the olive oil lightly over the bread.

4. Add one of the variations on 226-231 pages.

   a. Sprinkle selected herb or spice
   b. Spread topping
   c. Add more herb or spice as desired

5. Scatter (optional) the walnut pieces over the sandwich.

SANDWICH VARIATIONS

GREEN BEAN GOURMET SANDWICH

Makes an individual serving

The CR Way Essential Sandwich (pages 225–226) recipe Step 4:

Green Bean Gourmet Sandwich	
Calories:	202.78
Protein (g):	6.82
Carbohydrates (g):	15.12
Sugars (g):	2.61
Glucose (g):	0.02
Fructose (g):	0.01
Dietary Fiber (g):	14.51
Fat (g):	15.26
Saturated Fat (g):	1.58
Monounsaturated Fat (g):	5.91
Polyunsaturated Fat (g):	5.44
Omega-3 (g):	1.44
Omega-6 (g):	3.00
Phytosterols (mg):	5.45
Lutein+zeaxanthin (mcg):	24.44
Total Folate (mcg):	11.71
Tocopherol, Gamma (mg):	2.21
Calcium (mg):	17.75
Magnesium (mg):	26.50
Phosphorus (mg):	48.81
Potassium (mg):	348.21
Sodium (mg):	74.39
Copper (mg):	0.16
Iron (mg):	0.45
Manganese (mg):	0.40
Selenium (mcg):	1.32

a. ⅛ teaspoon ground ginger or to taste sprinkled on the Essential Sandwich

b. ½ to 1 container puréed organic green beans, Gerber Baby Food (50 to 100 gm), amount to meet preference and nutritional plan, spread on bread

c. Top with additional ground ginger and ground or whole flaxseed, as desired

SAVORY SALMON SANDWICH

Makes an individual serving

Essential Sandwich Recipe
(pages 225–226) Step 4:

a. ⅛ teaspoon ground ginger or dried dill, sprinkled on the bread, or to taste

b. 2 to 2½ ounces poached salmon or canned water-packed salmon, with bones and no salt added, spread on bread

c. Top with additional ground ginger or dill as desired

Savory Salmon Sandwich	
Calories:	199.75
Protein (g):	17.55
Carbohydrates (g):	4.0
Dietary Fiber (g):	8.35
Fat (g):	10.18
Saturated Fat (g):	1.66
Monounsaturated Fat (g):	4.47
Polyunsaturated Fat (g):	2.11
Omega-3 (g):	0.88
Omega-6 (g):	0.32
Vit-A (mcg_RAE):	37.54
Vit-B2 Riboflavin (mg):	0.66
Vit-B3 Niacin (mg):	4.78
Vit-B5 Pantothenic Acid (mg):	0.39
Vit-B6 Pyridoxine (mg):	0.25
Total Folate (mcg):	16.69
Vit-B12 Cyanocobalamin (mcg):	0.21
Calcium (mg):	171.14
Magnesium (mg):	46.80
Phosphorus (mg):	274.43
Potassium (mg):	349.26
Sodium (mg):	103.24
Copper (mg):	0.06
Iron (mg):	1.12
Selenium (mcg):	25.07
Zinc (mg):	1.00

MUSHROOM MAGIC SANDWICH

Makes an individual serving

Essential Sandwich Recipe
(pages 225-226) Step 4:

  a. 3½ ounces of the vegetables from Mushroom Magic Soup

  b. Use Mushroom Magic broth for extra moistening, if desired

Mushroom Magic Sandwich	
Calories:	137.21
Protein (g):	5.11
Carbohydrates (g):	14.40
Sugars (g):	2.77
Glucose (g):	0.27
Fructose (g):	0.16
Dietary Fiber (g):	12.15
Fat (g):	5.12
Saturated Fat (g):	0.51
Monounsaturated Fat (g):	2.51
Polyunsaturated Fat (g):	0.55
Phytosterols (mg):	4.23
Lutein+zeaxanthin (mcg):	1.28
Vit-B1 Thiamine (mg):	0.15
Vit-B2 Riboflavin (mg):	0.60
Vit-B3 Niacin (mg):	3.03
Vit-B5 Pantothenic Acid (mg):	0.55
Total Folate (mcg):	22.97
Vit-C (mg):	31.50
Vit-D (IU):	52.95
Tocopherol, Gamma (mg):	0.19
Calcium (mg):	25.46
Magnesium (mg):	41.81
Phosphorus (mg):	99.12
Potassium (mg):	394.68
Sodium (mg):	78.12
Copper (mg):	0.19
Iron (mg):	0.71
Manganese (mg):	0.15
Selenium (mcg):	3.53
Zinc (mg):	0.65

SAVORY SPINACH SANDWICH

Makes an individual serving

Essential Sandwich recipe
(pages 225-226) Step 4:

a. 3 ounces Savory Spinach
   (see recipe page 187-188)
b. Use spinach broth for extra
   moistening as desired

c. Garnish with 2 or 3 walnut
   halves, according to CR
   plan for fat intake

d. Garnish further with 1
   teaspoon or so of flaxseeds,
   according to fiber intake
   plan

Savory Spinach Sandwich	
Calories:	202.44
Protein (g):	8.13
Carbohydrates (g):	13.33
Sugars (g):	1.17
Glucose (g):	0.27
Fructose (g):	0.15
Dietary Fiber (g):	16.31
Fat (g):	15.53
Saturated Fat (g):	1.59
Monounsaturated Fat (g):	5.91
Polyunsaturated Fat (g):	5.46
Omega-3 (g):	1.44
Omega-6 (g):	3.00
Phytosterols (mg):	7.16
Lutein+zeaxanthin (mcg):	25.97
Vit-A IU:	4590.23
Vit-B1 Thiamine (mg):	0.10
Total Folate (mcg):	14.12
Vit-C (mg):	19.47
Tocopherol, Gamma (mg):	2.20
Calcium (mg):	87.63
Magnesium (mg):	28.20
Phosphorus (mg):	57.14
Potassium (mg):	218.59
Sodium (mg):	177.21
Copper (mg):	0.18
Iron (mg):	1.61
Manganese (mg):	0.41
Selenium (mcg):	1.79

VEGETABLE VISION SANDWICH

Makes an individual serving

Essential Sandwich recipe
(pages 225–226) Step 4:

    a. ⅛ teaspoon of herb or spice—ground ginger, oregano, garlic or your preference—sprinkled over sandwich

    b. 3½ ounces of boiled vegetables you have on hand, e.g., onions, peppers, green beans, broccoli, cauliflower, cabbage, kohlrabi, turnip, celery root (see Foods to Choose for more) Broth reserved from vegetables for extra moistening as desired

    c. Top with sprinkling of the herb or spice used on the base, as desired

Vegetable Vision Sandwich	
Calories:	210.66
Protein (g):	7.15
Carbohydrates (g):	18.03
Sugars (g):	5.09
Glucose (g):	2.07
Fructose (g):	1.23
Dietary Fiber (g):	13.87
Fat (g):	15.44
Saturated Fat (g):	1.61
Monounsaturated Fat (g):	5.94
Polyunsaturated Fat (g):	5.51
Omega-3 (g):	1.45
Omega-6 (g):	3.07
Phytosterols (mg):	23.13
Carotene, beta (mcg):	2.17
Lutein+zeaxanthin (mcg):	28.41
Vit-B1 Thiamine (mg):	0.13
Total Folate (mcg):	26.51
Vit-C (mg):	8.99
Tocopherol, Gamma (mg):	2.20
Calcium (mg):	39.32
Magnesium (mg):	37.00
Phosphorus (mg):	83.21
Potassium (mg):	339.90
Sodium (mg):	72.30
Copper (mg):	0.23
Manganese (mg):	0.49
Selenium (mcg):	1.83

DELIGHTFUL DESSERTS

All desserts here are individual servings—which can easily be doubled, tripled, etc., as desired.

DESSERT SANDWICH

Makes an individual serving

Essential Sandwich recipe
(pages 225–226) Step 4:

a. ¼ teaspoon pumpkin pie spice or ground ginger, nutmeg, cloves, and cinnamon, sprinkled over bread, or to taste

b. Broth if crust needs moistening

c. Cut into small bites to savor the flavor

Dessert Sandwich	
Calories:	168.45
Protein (g):	5.82
Carbohydrates (g):	8.25
Sugars (g):	0.63
Glucose (g):	0.02
Fructose (g):	0.01
Dietary Fiber (g):	12.54
Fat (g):	15.30
Saturated Fat (g):	1.61
Monounsaturated Fat (g):	5.91
Polyunsaturated Fat (g):	5.44
Omega-3 (g):	1.44
Omega-6 (g):	3.00
Phytosterols (mg):	5.57
Stigmasterol (mg):	0.07
Lutein+zeaxanthin (mcg):	25.25
Total Folate (mcg):	11.84
Tocopherol, Gamma (mg):	2.20
Calcium (mg):	20.38
Magnesium (mg):	26.66
Phosphorus (mg):	48.98
Potassium (mg):	178.01
Sodium (mg):	69.54
Copper (mg):	0.16
Iron (mg):	0.51
Manganese (mg):	0.40
Selenium (mcg):	1.28

BERRIES AND WHEAT BERRIES

Makes an individual serving

Using the Wheat Berry Cereal as a dessert works beautifully. A smaller serving is often enough, for example:

- 2½ ounces Sweet Wheat Berries (70 gm)
- 2½ ounces thawed berries (70 gm)
- 2 teaspoons (rounded) lecithin granules (5 gm)
- 2 or 3 walnut halves, ground or broken (5 gm)
- 2 teaspoons lemon juice (10 gm), or to taste

VERY BERRY DESSERT

Thaw the berries in the refrigerator as close to serving time as practicable. It is fine if they are still a bit frozen—it may remind you of ice cream. Using fresh, local berries is, of course, also fine. Any of the other berries, as well as mixed berries, can be substituted for wild blueberries.

Berries and Wheat Berries	
Calories:	177.57
Protein (g):	3.72
Carbohydrates (g):	29.55
Sugars (g):	4.99
Sucrose (g):	0.12
Dietary Fiber (g):	3.69
Fat (g):	6.09
Saturated Fat (g):	1.00
Monounsaturated Fat (g):	1.31
Polyunsaturated Fat (g):	3.77
Omega-3 (g):	0.45
Omega-6 (g):	1.90
Phytosterols (mg):	3.60
Vit-B1 Thiamine (mg):	0.28
Vit-B2 Riboflavin (mg):	0.10
Vit-B3 Niacin (mg):	4.26
Vit-B5 Pantothenic Acid (mg):	0.85
Vit-B6 Pyridoxine (mg):	0.29
Total Folate (mcg):	20.65
Vit-C (mg):	43.80
Tocopherol, Gamma (mg):	1.04
Vit-K (mcg):	22.63
Calcium (mg):	27.55
Magnesium (mg):	7.90
Phosphorus (mg):	161.69
Potassium (mg):	114.00
Sodium (mg):	0.52
Chromium (mcg):	0.30
Copper (mg):	0.15
Iodine (mcg):	0.68
Iron (mg):	1.60
Manganese (mg):	1.07
Selenium (mcg):	1.26

Makes an individual serving

2 ½ ounces frozen (or fresh) organic
wild blueberries or other berries
(70 gm)

2 teaspoons (4 gm) soy lecithin granules

2 to 3 (5 gm) walnut halves

5 gm lemon juice, or to taste

1. Place the berries in a side
   dish.

2. Sprinkle the lecithin over
   the berries.

3. Break the walnut halves
   into pieces and add to the
   berries.

4. Stir and serve.

Very Berry Dessert	
Calories:	218.41
Protein (g):	1.05
Carbohydrates (g):	10.11
Sugars (g):	3.56
Sucrose (g):	0.12
Dietary Fiber (g):	2.05
Fat (g):	19.26
Saturated Fat (g):	4.31
Monounsaturated Fat (g):	4.45
Polyunsaturated Fat (g):	10.36
Omega-3 (g):	0.45
Omega-6 (g):	1.90
Phytosterols (mg):	3.60
Vit-C (mg):	30.92
Tocopherol, Gamma (mg):	1.04
Calcium (mg):	16.33
Phosphorus (mg):	477.30
Potassium (mg):	382.05
Sodium (mg):	0.10

WHAT'S GOING ON?
YOU LOOK YOUNGER!

As we come to the end of this book, we are getting ready to take our evening walk. It's a very special time we share. We have spent a lot of our walks over the past year talking about you—thinking about how best to share this lifestyle. We hope that the ideas here will help you realize your full potential for health, happiness, and long life. Do be prepared! You may notice that people will begin to say, "Gee, you look terrific—younger than when we saw you last." We wish we could be there to see the delight in your eyes. Congratulations—you are on *The CR Way*!

Wishing you much health and happiness,

Paul and Meredith

PART IV

APPENDICES

Appendix A: CR Groundbreakers

Appendix B: Resveratrol

Appendix C: Suggested Lab Tests

Appendix D: Frequently Asked Questions

Appendix E: Glossary

Appendix F: Bibliography

APPENDIX A

CR GROUNDBREAKERS

The calorie restriction science presented in *The CR Way* provides the essential knowledge for you to begin your journey. But breakthrough research continues daily, however, and we encourage you to continue your exploration by learning to use PubMed.gov, Google Scholar, MedlinePlus.gov, Mendosa.com, and other information resources and by joining the Calorie Restriction Society (www.calorierestriction.org). All of these resources will give you updates and help provide the depth of understanding necessary to make objective choices. Using these resources will give you constant input from the best scientists in the world. You, no doubt, noticed the PMIDs in many of the citations, included to facilitate your finding these references.

Here is a guide to some of the groundbreaking scientists who have influenced us along with thousands of other CR practitioners:

STEPHEN AUSTAD, PH.D.: Deepened our understanding of the relationship of growth to aging, helping us remain wary of growth-stimulating practices that may actually accelerate aging.

ANDY BRAWLEY, PH.D., and RICHARD LORD, PH.D., of Metametrix Laboratories: gave us new insights into how nutrition affects health at the molecular level—ultimately helping us better evaluate how well our CR practice is working.

HAIM COHEN, PH.D., of the Sinclair Lab: demonstrated the relationship between the insulin/IGF-I pathway and the energy-sensitive SIRT1—helping us focus on aspects of CR that can really make a difference in how fast we age.

BRIAN DELANEY: Was a principal founder and developer of the Calorie Restriction Society, which provides valuable information on all aspects of CR and longevity. We've improved many of our lifestyle practices based on input from Society members.

LUIGI FONTANA, M.D., PH.D.: Created the first human studies on CR—providing a standard to judge our CR practice and valuable guidance on how to safely live a CR life.

LIVIA GAN, PH.D.: Demonstrated the relationship between SIRT1 activity and IGFBP1—giving us a means to test for SIRT1 activation clinically.

LEONARD GUARENTE, PH.D.: Heads the lab that discovered the function of SIR2 in aging—ultimately influencing how we plan our CR lifestyle.

WEI GU, PH.D.: Discovered the relationship between the cancer protector p53 and SIRT1—influencing us to moderate cell-proliferating activities when our SIRT1 gene is likely to be expressed.

JOHN HOLLOSZY, PH.D.: Deepened our understanding of the role exercise plays in health and its limitation in slowing aging—resulting in our moderation of the amount of exercise we do each day.

SHIN IMAI, M.D., PH.D.: Helped us understand the relationship between SIRT1 and NAD—reinforcing the importance of keeping glucose low as part of the best way to practice CR.

CYNTHIA KENYON, PH.D.: Discovered the important inflence of the insulin–IGF-I system on aging—leading us to eliminate foods that provoke insulin, independent of calories.

ED MASORO, PH.D.: His prolific writing gave us tools to understand CR physiology—helping us avoid lifestyle practices that counter our CR benefits.

MARK MATTSON, PH.D.: Discovered that time away from food is important for producing CR-related benefits, especially cognitive improvements—influencing us to include a significant daily fasting period in our regimen.

MARTY MAYO, PH.D.: Demonstrated that activating SIRT1 also controls a central driver of inflammation, NF-kappaB—resulting in our paying close attention to how to prevent activation of inflammation pathways.

CLIVE MCKAY, M.D.: Did the first major calorie restriction research on laboratory animals—sixty years later we began our CR practice.

PERE PUIGSERVER, PH.D.: Discovered SIRT1's link to gluconeogenesis—helping us understand the importance of glucose control for longevity.

DAVID SINCLAIR, PH.D.: Helped us understand the pathways that must be activated for SIRT1 to be expressed. His work on resveratrol is a leap forward in how a CR mimetic may be used for better health.

STEPHEN SPINDLER, PH.D.: Especially renowned for genetic microarray work on calorie-restricted animals, helped us understand that CR benefits can be quickly activated at any age.

TED (THEODORE B.) VANITALLIE, M.D.: Helped us understand the health benefits of ketones—influencing us to make ketones part of our CR practice.

HELEN VLASSARA, M.D.: Her in-depth research into advanced glycation endproducts influenced us to prepare foods in ways that minimize exposure to AGE.

ROY WALFORD, M.D.: His books and software helped us begin to live a CR lifestyle. His daughter Lisa continues his work.

RICK WEINDRUCH, PH.D.: Wrote the first CR article that we read, showing us how humans could practice CR.

APPENDIX B

RESVERATROL

Like any lifestyle change, embracing *The CR Way* takes time, effort, and commitment. The health benefits are certainly worth it.

Still, most of us wish at one time or another for that magic bullet: a simple pill that would safely and effectively reduce the effects of aging; prevent cancer, heart disease, and diabetes; increase memory, and extend life, and all without having to count calories.

The magic bullet may have been found when David Sinclair at Harvard University and his colleagues demonstrated that resveratrol, a chemical found in plants, mimics the effects of CR. Just as limiting calories triggers the low-level stress response—hormesis—which, in turn, jump-starts the SIRT1 longevity gene, resveratrol mimics this stress, activating SIRT1.

For years many CR researchers have stated that they hope calorie restriction science will lead to the development of calorie restriction mimetics, that is, drugs that mimic the health and longevity benefits of calorie restriction without the need to limit calories. Now resveratrol has emerged as the leading candidate for the mimetic many hoped for. The key to resveratrol benefits is that it activates the same longevity genes and cell-signaling pattern as calorie restriction.

Metformin, a drug used to treat diabetes, has also been tested as a CR mimetic and has been shown to produce some longevity effects. However, the primary effect of metformin is lowering glucose levels—a benefit that can be achieved naturally through *The CR Way*.

What has excited the scientific community is the research showing that resveratrol may not only provide the same benefits as CR without restricting calories, but it may also, in fact, counteract the damaging effects of high-calorie diets. In the latest study by Dr. Sinclair's lab and the National Institute on Aging, a group of mice was fed a diet consisting of 60 percent fat, which, unsurprisingly, caused weight gain, symptoms of diabetes, and early death. Another group of mice was fed the same diet but was given resveratrol. Although they gained as much weight as the control group, these mice showed no signs of the elevated glucose and insulin levels that would indicate diabetes.

Even more fascinating was that the resveratrol mice actually improved their motor skills as they aged. This parallels our own discovery of enhanced cognitive capabilities on CR.

The work at Harvard has generated worldwide interest—prompting many labs to do related research and increasing sales of resveratrol supplements. Already several studies have demonstrated a broad range of potential benefits, including:

Cardiovascular Health—inhibits blood clotting, helps prevent atherosclerosis, and inhibits heart-aging inflammation.

Cancer—inhibits cell proliferation of a variety of human cancer cell lines, including breast, prostate, stomach, colon, pancreatic and thyroid cancers. Animal experiments have shown significant inhibition of esophageal, intestinal, and breast cancers.

Diabetes—The first clinical trials of Sirtris Pharmaceuticals are focusing on **SRT501**, an improved resveratrol molecule for control of glucose and improved insulin secretion. This builds on the most readily demonstrable benefit of resveratrol in humans—glucose control, an integral part of *The CR Way*.

With such promising benefits, should health-minded people drink red wine or eat resveratrol-containing foods? The chances are slim that the amount obtained will have any effect. Some red wine may contain small amounts of resveratrol, as do grapes, raspberries, peanuts, and numerous other plants. However, to gain the amount of resveratrol comparable to what is used in laboratory experiments, you would have to drink or eat far more than is healthy, wise, or even possible.

Normal servings of foods containing resveratrol are not close to the amounts used for resveratrol research. The Harvard study that extended the life of overweight mice used 22.4 milligrams per kilogram of body weight. For a 160-pound male, that translates into a megadose of 1,575 milligrams.

Since obtaining resveratrol in wine or foods is not easily possible, why not just pop a resveratrol supplement? It is certainly seductive.

The best way we can answer the question about whether to take resveratrol or not is to provide you with the knowledge to make your own decision. Such knowledge will empower you to make objective decisions about resveratrol and other supplements that come along.

BASIC INFORMATION

These days most resveratrol for supplements is extracted from knotweed, a shrublike plant also known as known as *Polygonum cuspidatum*. Resveratrol has been approved by the Environmental Protection Agency as nontoxic. It is not recommended for pregnant women or growing children. Resveratrol can be either trans-resveratrol—the biologically active form of the molecule—or cis-resveratrol—a form that does not activate the SIRT1 gene. Exposure to light can change trans-resveratrol to the cis-form. To be effective, resveratrol must be protected from light, heat, and oxygen during manufacture and subsequently when stored.

The key to obtaining benefits from resveratrol is finding a reliable supplement company that supplies resveratrol that is biologically active. Supplements are not regulated like pharmaceuticals, so some products provide no more effect than a placebo. You can gauge possible biological activity by using a glucose meter to test the resveratrol supplement's effect on the blood glucose increase caused by a meal. If a noticeable lowering is achieved, at least it is producing some beneficial effect.

Another consideration is how much to take. No one knows the true answer to this question. Some manufacturers provide 20 milligrams per capsule. However, a top resveratrol producer currently provides 100 milligrams per capsule. So, every label must be read.

Always remember that the effect of anything may be greater for CR practitioners who eat limited quantities of food. Advice from a leading pharmacology expert who also follows a calorie-restricted diet is to start with as small a dose as possible and test it carefully before increasing the dosage. Most important, always listen to your body. If you notice something out of the ordinary, like extra fatigue, you may be taking too much. Cutting back or starting over would be a good idea.

Use *The CR Way* effectiveness panel (Chapter 8) to test any new supplement or lifestyle change. These markers provide a good indication of just how well your CR program is working to slow aging. Resveratrol or any other supplement you add to your life should produce improvements in these parameters.

ALWAYS CHECK WITH YOUR DOCTOR

Supplements and medications must be processed by the liver. As it turns out, resveratrol affects a liver enzyme complex (CYP1) that is responsible for metabolizing many medications and some common substances, including caffeine and theophylline, a stimulant in tea.

So, before taking resveratrol it is important to ask your doctor if you are taking a drug, vitamin, or herb, etc., that is processed by CYP1.

SUGGESTED LAB TESTS

The following tests will be done either in your doctor's office or by prescription at a nearby clinical lab. If you look back at the results of the CR cohort of the Washington University studies (page 148), you will see goals that are worthy of your effort. Keep in mind that the subjects in the cohort had all been practicing CR for at lest six years, so these numbers really are goals and not to be discouraging if you are not there yet. If you need a reminder about the tests' units of measure, you'll find them in the Glossary, on page 269, Lab Test Units of Measure.

TOTAL CHOLESTEROL, mg/dl, Cholesterol is a fatlike substance made by the bodies of humans and other animals. A total cholesterol test includes measures of several types of blood fats, including LDL-C, HDL-C, and triglycerides.

LDL-C, mg/dl, Low-Density Lipoprotein-Cholesterol is the kind of cholesterol that, while essential to human life, increases the plaque deposited inside the arteries and raises the risk of athero-sclerosis.

HDL-C (HIGH-DENSITY LIPOPROTEIN-CHOLESTEROL), mg/dl, The kind of cholesterol that helps carry fat away from artery walls.

TOTAL CHOL:HDL-C RATIO The ratio of total cholesterol to HDL is important; the smaller the number, the better. For example, some-one with a total cholesterol of 200 and an HDL of 60 would have a cholesterol-to-HDL ratio of 3.3 (200÷60=3.3). If instead, that person's HDL were low—let's say 35—the total cholesterol-to-HDL ratio would be higher: 5.7.

TRIGLYCERIDES, mg/dl The most common type of fat in food and in the human body, where it is also made. Excess triglycerides are stored in adipose tissue and are used to provide energy. High levels in the blood are often found in people who have high blood cholesterol or heart problems, or are overweight or have diabetes. High blood levels also increase the chances of developing athero-sclerosis.

SYSTOLIC BP, mmHg The Blood Pressure of the systole—the con-traction of the heart by which the blood is forced onward and the circulation is kept up. It is the first and the higher of the two blood pressure numbers.

DIASTOLIC BP, mmHg The Blood Pressure of the diastole—the dilation or passive rhythmical expansion of the cavities of the heart during which they fill with blood. It is the second and the lower of the two blood pressure numbers.

FASTING GLUCOSE, mg/dl The level of glucose in the blood after a period of time without food, the body's baseline level when the effect of food is absent (usually overnight, lab requirements vary).

FASTING INSULIN (microIU or µIU/ml) The level of insulin in the blood after a period of time without food (usually overnight, lab requirements vary).

T3 (ng/dl) This thyroid hormone feeds back to the hypothalamus and pituitary gland to regulate the release of both TSH and TRH (Thyroid Releasing Hormone, which stimulates the release of TSH).

hs-CRP (mg/L) High sensitivity C-reactive protein—sensitive indicator of inflammation status and predictor of heart attack risk.

TNF-α (pg/ml) Tumor Necrosis Factor-alpha—compounds in the blood, produced by activated macrophages and other mononuclear leukocytes—both of which are signs of the mammalian immune system's going on the defensive against some "intruder." TNF-α has a deadly effect against tumor cells, and research shows it to increase the ability to reject tumor transplants in laboratory animals.

TGF-β1 Transforming Growth Factor—TGF-β exists as several subtypes, all of which are found in hematopoietic tissue (tissue in which blood or blood cells are formed), stimulate wound healing, and, in vitro, are antagonists of lymph cell formation and of the formation of bone marrow or the cells arising from it. TGF-β is a factor synthesized in a wide variety of tissues. The transforming growth factor beta1 (TGF-β1) plays a key role in regulating tissue repair and remodeling after injury.

HRest Heart Rate at rest—in general a lower number is better.

IGF-I Insulin-like Growth Factor-I (somatomedin), measured in ng (nanograms) per milliliter of blood—a protein hormone produced primarily by the liver in response to human growth hormone (hGH). It plays a role in helping hGH cause changes in cells that lead to growth.

FREQUENTLY ASKED QUESTIONS

Based on the extensive media interviews and CR conferences we have conducted over the years, the give-and-take of a Q & A session invariably draws out interesting questions we may not have previously addressed. Following are some of the most commonly asked questions along with our answers. It also provides a quick index for points of interest to return to again and again.

Q: How do you handle hunger? Do you eat frequent small meals, snack between meals, or what?

A: We accept occasional hunger as part of this lifestyle. The hunger sensation is not extreme, and it makes us glad: To be more likely to attain our health and longevity goals, we intend to eat less than our bodies might crave, so hunger is a signal that we are doing what we intend. We definitely like it better than the bloated feeling of being satiated. Another cause for joy is that when the body is fed fewer calories than it "expects," it goes looking for more. That takes the form of the cells' digesting matter that they "didn't bother with before." This results in a cleanup, a sort of cellular level detox. We love it! Our bodies are so smart.

Q: How do you maintain a low weight, yet still consume enough calories to sustain an exercise program?

A: As your body adapts to CR, you begin to burn fewer calories per day, while your energy increases. That's a perfect combination for having the energy you need for moderate exercise. A large part of calorie restriction is keeping a close eye on your caloric intake so that you not only do not take in too many, but also so you don't take in too few. A daily intake of 1,900 calories is plenty for Paul, for example, to sustain his weight at his level of exercise activity. He weighs himself regularly, and if his weight slips lower than his target of 137, he increases his caloric intake until his weight is stable.

Q: I run about seventy miles per month and lift weights regularly. While the CR lifestyle appeals to me, I don't think I would be consuming enough calories to remain strong while exercising.

A: There are many levels of CR, so it's not necessary to restrict calories the way we do to get some benefits. Studies show that CR gives far more longevity benefits than exercise, though, so we personally follow a moderate exercise program—making it easier to sustain our limited calorie intake.

Exercise is recommended in moderation rather than the high level of activity you refer to. On a daily basis we exercise moderately (run and walk) and twice a week more vigorously for weight training.

Q: What kinds of foods do you eat to maintain good health and do these foods satisfy hunger?

A: We eat nutrient-dense foods, such as salmon and lentils and carbs with low to moderate glycemic rankings (cabbage, broccoli, collards, sweet potatoes, and the like), as well as fruit (blueberries and strawberries, for example) and fats (walnuts and olive oil, etc.). In addition to being loaded with nutrients, the phytochemicals in many of these foods provide extra health benefits such as protection against certain cancers.

The high fiber in *The CR Way* diet helps satisfy hunger.

Q: While on this diet, did you experience any light-headedness or dizziness? Did you feel more tired than usual?

A: We have been living this healthful lifestyle for fourteen years. We have not experienced any light-headedness or dizziness. Rather than feeling more tired, we have more energy. Yes, weight loss is virtually universally experienced when fewer calories are consumed than the body would normally use. And we're talking about a 20 percent reduction in intake. If you are interested in more detail, the Calorie Restriction Society is an organization of people, most of whom are CR practitioners, who exchange information about the process and how it works (http://www.calorierestriction.org/).

Q: Do you lose any muscle mass on CR?

A: This is different for different people, but we have gained muscle mass because we exercise with that in mind: For maximum strength training, exercise each muscle group only twice per week, which is enough to provoke significant strength gains. True, we might have gained more muscle if we were not on CR, but our fitness goal is optimal function, not muscle size.

Q: How does CR affect a person's mental abilities? Does it slow you down, making concentration and problem solving more difficult?

A: There are many different ways to approach CR. Our experience has been tremendous improvement in mental capabilities. Some of the most dramatic improvement came when we integrated Daily Limited Fasting into our CR regimen, so that in addition to limiting calories, we also spend a significant time away from food—finishing our last food of the day, at say, 1:00 p.m. and not eating again until 6:00 or 7:00 the next morning. We continue to work productively during that period and have found our energy and intellectual sharpness has actually improved while on CR. Exciting research by Mark P. Mattson, at the NIA (National Institute on Aging) labs, has shown that such fasting provokes the secretion of neuroprotective chemicals involved in protecting and regenerating brain cells.

Q: What's the difference between calorie restriction and semistarvation?

A: Semistarvation is depriving your body of what it needs. We give our bodies what they need to function optimally. Our interest is to nourish ourselves as close to the optimal as we can, using foods that are delicious. We measure our food intake, track the components, and experiment with spicing. We eat proteins and fats relatively sparingly, and it does take a lot of nutrient-dense vegetables and fruit to add up to enough calories even for us. We should rush to assure you that this attention to detail is not necessary to gain real benefits from CR. Optimal health-and-nutrition is our passion, and you will find almost as many versions of CR practice as there are practitioners. The Calorie Restriction Society is a good place to learn more is (http://www.calorie-restriction.org/).

Q: Is calorie restriction all right for teenagers who want to be healthy but still want to eat fewer calories and lose weight?

A: The research is not yet definitive on how early it is advantageous or safe for a person to begin CR. So while it is probably good for

everyone to eat in moderation, one should be careful about restricting calories during the teen years when the body is still growing. We would recommend that everyone include high-quality
nutrient-dense foods in their diet like sweet potatoes, broccoli, and
other yummies that offer benefits at any age.

Q: How quickly will I see results on *The CR Way*?

A: We recommend starting out slowly and gradually, even as simply
as realigning the foods you eat to maximize nutrition without cutting calories. As your body becomes acclimated, you can gradually
reduce caloric intake, while maintaining the nutrient-dense calories. You will begin to notice changes in your body—not only in
weight loss, but a general feeling of health and well-being. By following *The CR Way*, the combination of foods, meditation, fasting,
and exercise will work together to greatly enhance your life. But
remember, gradually is the safest way. Try to integrate the dietary
changes into your lifestyle over a period of a year or more.

Q: Would a vegetarian or vegan diet be feasible?

A: Because *The CR Way* emphasizes nutrient-dense food over empty
calories, vegetarian and vegan diets are most certainly feasible. Vegetables, nuts, grains, and beans are staples in our own daily menu,
and although we are not strict vegetarians, we rarely eat meat. Our
dietary practices also include an effort to control glucose, paying
atention to the Glycemic Index of foods. We are currently eating
less protein than we used to because research shows that protein
restriction has similar effects to calorie restriction. A vegan diet is
very possible, and many members of the Calorie Restriction Society
are vegans. Our particular approach does include small amounts of
animal protein: salmon and eggs, for example.

Q: What is meant by "extreme caloric restriction"? Some definitions put it at 15 percent to 20 percent lower than the weight you were at when you were in your twenties. How much must you reduce your caloric intake to achieve this?

A: We are serious calorie restrictors but not extreme. Our caloric intake is about 20 percent reduced from that of an average person for our heights. Probably, national averages are too high anyway because so much of our society suffers from obesity. CR is not really about losing weight, but rather it's about maintaining a comfortable weight where you can eat the fewest calories. If you get too slim, you will actually need more calories to maintain your weight than if your weight loss is moderate. Our favorite calorie restrictor, Ralph, lived to 104 at 5 feet 10 inches and 148 pounds. Toward the end of his life, he ate only 600 to 800 calories a day, but he *maintained his weight* with that small caloric intake. We always recommend losing weight slowly and when you find you can maintain a weight that allows you to restrict calories at 20 percent of normal for your height, it's probably best to stop there.

Q: How do I go about getting the nutrients that I need and how do I know I am getting the right amount while doing CR?

A: Track your nutrition intake with a software package designed for that purpose. By doing so, you will learn a great deal about choosing the best foods and the right amounts for you. NutriBase Nutrition and Fitness Software (NutriBase.com) is some of the best.

Q: What are the top five vegetables to eat with the least calories and most nutrients?

A: Spinach, collards, kale, broccoli, and turnip greens are our favorites for low calories and high nutrients. Lightly steamed sweet potatoes, a bit higher in calories, are another nutrient-dense favorite. Lots of other veggies are excellent. Which ones we want to eat, when, and in what amount depends on whether we are looking for something to support our immune systems, whether we are looking for more fiber or less, what other nutrients we've had that day, and of course which wonderful flavors we want to enjoy.

Q: I get weak and shaky if I don't eat carbohydrates. How do you have the energy to get anything done and not feel hungry all of the time? What is the secret? Are you taking certain supplements to help with the food reduction?

A: Our blood sugar is on the low side—in the 80s or 90s after meals and in the 70s after fasting overnight. Note that because our bodies have adapted to these lowered glucose levels we rarely have the weak or shaky feelings that many people experience with lower blood sugar. We select foods that rank low on the Glycemic Index, like salmon, lightly boiled sweet potatoes, and cauliflower, that provide a slow, steady source of glucose when digested. We avoid foods like white potatoes that provide a rapid influx of glucose into the bloodstream. For a thorough list of foods and their glycemic ratings, as well as in-depth info on this subject, log on to David Mendosa's Web site (http://www.mendosa.com/). This definitely is working for us. We feel better in general. No supplements are necessary to help food reduction produce these extraordinary benefits.

Q: Do you eat the traditional three meals a day or small meals frequently throughout the day?

A: We space the courses out so that we can get the effect we want. We are following (at: www.Pubmed.gov) the research of

Mark P. Mattson, at NIA in Bethesda, Maryland, with great interest. His work shows that the body's time away from food may be as important as the reduced amount of food. Therefore, we are timing our meals so that we have about fifteen to seventeen hours between our last meal of the day and breakfast.

GLOSSARY

ACID: Traditionally considered any chemical compound that when dissolved in water gives a solution with a pH less than 7.0.

ADVANCED GLYCATION ENDPRODUCTS (AGE): A group of molecules formed inside the body when sugars combine with proteins, lipids, and nucleic acids. AGEs are often formed by cooking.

ALKALINE: Any chemical compound that when dissolved in water gives a pH above 7.0.

ARTERIAL INTIMA-MEDIA THICKNESS: The thickness of the inner and middle layers of arteries, in particular of the carotid artery in the neck. Thickening of the arterial intima-media is a marker for atherosclerosis and is used to predict coronary artery disease.

ATHEROSCLEROSIS: A condition in which fatty material collects along the walls of arteries. This plaque thickens, hardens, and may eventually block the arteries. It is one of several types of arteriosclerosis.

BASELINE: Used on *The CR Way* to refer to the fasting level of glucose as well as other biomarkers—where you start. The baseline serves as a reference point to gauge future test results.

BENFOTIAMINE: A highly absorbable form of vitamin B-1 that may inhibit the formation of advanced glycation endproducts.

BIFIDOBACTERIA: A bacterial group that exerts health-promoting properties within the human gut. Bifidobacteria aid in digestion, are associated with a lower incidence of allergies, and also prevent some forms of tumor growth. Some bifidobacteria are being used as probiotics, which are supplements of microorganisms that have a beneficial effect on gut health.

BIOMARKERS: Cellular or molecular indicators of exposure, disease, or susceptibility to disease. Biological changes that characterize the aging process—measurable through lab tests.

BMI—BODY MASS INDEX: A number that shows the relationship of a person's weight to height. It is commonly used to classify obesity, overweight, and underweight in adults. You can check your BMI by referring to the chart on page 116.

BRAIN-DERIVED NEUROTROPHIC: FACTOR, OR BDNF: A regulator of neuronal growth, survival, and function (during development and in the adult brain).

BRAN—*See* GRAIN.

CALORIE—A UNIT OF FOOD ENERGY: In nutrition terms, the word "calorie" is used instead of the more precise scientific term, "kilocalorie," which represents the amount of energy required to raise the temperature of a gram of water one degree centigrade at sea level.

CANCER: Any malignant growth or tumor caused by abnormal and uncontrolled cell division; it may spread to other parts of the body through the lymphatic system or the bloodstream.

CARBOHYDRATE: One of the three main nutrients in food. Includes sugars, starches, celluloses, and gums, which are used as sources of energy by the body.

CARCINOGEN: A substance that give rise to malignant new growth (tumors) made up of epithelial cells tending to infiltrate the surrounding tissues and give rise to metastases. Carcinogen is widely used in the more general sense as any substance that causes cancer. In this sense, carcinogens reach us through air, water, and food. Careful selection of pure water, whole foods from organic sources, filters, and enforced clean-air and clean-water regulations reduce our exposure to these environmental dangers.

CAROTID ARTERY: Blood vessel that supplies the head and neck with oxygenated blood.

CELL SIGNALING: Communication among cells: any of several ways in which living cells of an organism communicate with one another—whether by direct contact between cells or by means of chemical signals carried by neurotransmitter substances, hormones, and messenger molecules.

CENTERING MEDITATION: A relaxing method of contemplation that replaces the thoughts, which usually occupy the mind, with a single meaningful word or phrase.

CEPHALIC PHASE INSULIN RELEASE: Insulin production thought to be provoked by the sight, smell, and taste of food (before any nutrient is absorbed).

CHOLESTEROL: A soft waxy substance manufactured by the liver and other organs and consumed as animal fat. Cholesterol is used in the manufacture of hormones, bile acid, and vitamin D. It is present in all parts of the body, including the nervous system, muscle, skin, liver, intestines, and heart. (*See also* SUGGESTED LAB TESTS in Appendix C, pages 247-248.)

DAILY LIMITED FASTING: Daily fasting for a period of time, usually overnight.

DHEA: Dehydroepiandrosterone is an important natural steroid produced by the adrenal glands, which are found atop the human kidneys. It is also produced in small quantities in the testis and the ovary. DHEA can be converted to several sex hormones, both male and female.

DIASTOLE: The part of the heart cycle when the heart muscle (myocardium) relaxes and expands: during diastole blood fills the heart chambers. Diastolic blood pressure measures the pressure on blood vessels walls when the heart is at rest. It is the second of the two blood pressure numbers.

DHA DOCOSAHEXAENOIC ACID: An omega-3 fatty acid that belongs to the class of nutrients called "essential fatty acids." It is found in fish oils of herring, mackerel, salmon, and sardines. It is also found in human breast milk.

DNA DEOXYRIBONUCLEIC ACID: Molecules inside cells that contain the genetic instructions for the formation and function of an organism. DNA carries the hereditary information that is passed on from one generation to the next.

DRI—DIETARY REFERENCE INTAKES: Development of the Dietary Reference Intakes under the auspices of the Food and Nutrition Board of the Institute of Medicine is a major revision of our nutrient and energy standards. DRI is a generic term for several new types of advisory reference values:

EAR—The Estimated Average Requirement is the nutrient intake estimated to meet the requirement defined by a specified indicator of adequacy in 50 percent of an age- and gender-specific group. At this level of intake, the remaining 50 percent of the specified group would not have met its needs.

RDA—The Recommended Dietary Allowance is the dietary intake level that is sufficient to meet the nutrient requirements of nearly all (97 to 98 percent) healthy individuals in a particular life stage and gender group.

AI—The Adequate Intake is a recommended intake value based on observed or experimentally determined approximations or estimates of nutrient intake by a group (or groups) of healthy people that are assumed to be adequate or used when an RDA cannot be determined.

UL—The tolerable Upper Intake Level is the highest level of daily nutrient intake that is likely to pose no risk of adverse health effects for almost all of the individuals in the general population. As intake increases above the UL, the risk of adverse effects increases.

DRI REPORTS: Have been published by the National Academies Press. This link presents their catalog: http://www.nap.edu/catalog/

11537.html. An extremely helpful quick-reference document that is available by PDF download is available from the IOM—the Institute of Medicine—at: http://www.iom.edu/Object.File/Master/21/372/0.pdf. Further, the National Agriculture Library's Web site makes the Food and Nutrition Information Center's documentation (including DRI Tables and Guidelines) very accessible at: http://fnic.nal.usda.gov/nal, using the following path: Home/Dietary Guidance/Dietary Reference Intakes/DRI Tables.

EFAS—ESSENTIAL FATTY ACIDS—*See* OMEGA FATTY ACIDS.

ENDOSPERM—*See* GRAIN.

EPA—EICOSAPENTAENOIC ACID: An omega-3 fatty acid that belongs to the class of nutrients known as essential fatty acids. It is found in fish oils of cod liver, herring, mackerel, salmon, and sardines. It is also found in human breast milk.

EPINEPHRINE: A hormone secreted by the adrenal gland that is released into the bloodstream in response to physical or mental stress, as from fear or injury. It initiates many bodily responses, including the stimulation of heart action and an increase in blood pressure, metabolic rate, and blood-glucose concentration. Also called "adrenaline."

ESTROGEN(S): The female hormones produced primarily by the ovaries. These steroid compounds induce menstruation and stimulate the development of secondary sexual characteristics in women. Estrogen is important for the maintenance of normal brain function and development of nerve cells. Small amounts of estrogen are also produced in men by the testes.

EVO—EXTRA VIRGIN OLIVE OIL: This is the purest form available from the olive oil processing. Choosing organic EVO provides an additional level of purity.

FAT: One of the three main nutrients in food, this type of caloric energy is essential for a variety of body functions, including organ protection, hormone balances, and a long-lasting fuel source for low-intensity exercise. Dietary fats are classified as saturated (animal flesh, butter, margarine, processed and fried foods) and unsaturated (vegetable oils). Unsaturated fats are the preferred food for health reasons.

FIBER: Parts of fruits and vegetables that cannot be digested—also called "bulk" or "roughage." Fiber, both soluble and insoluble, is an important component of a healthful diet and may play a role in preventing cancer and heart disease.

FREE RADICALS: Highly reactive molecules capable of causing tissue damage. Free radicals are common by-products of normal chemical reactions occurring in cells. The body has several mechanisms to deactivate free radicals. (*See also* REACTIVE OXYGEN MOLECULES.)

FRUCTOSE: A type of sugar found in many fruits and vegetables and in honey.

FUNCTIONAL FOOD: Food or food ingredient that has been shown to affect specific functions or systems in the body. Functional foods play an important role in disease prevention.

GALACTOSE: A sugar found in dairy products, beets, and gums.

GENE: The portion of DNA that directs the synthesis of amino acids that form proteins with highly specific functions.

GERM—*See* **GRAIN**.

GHRELIN (GHR): The hunger hormone, produced by epithelial cells of the stomach, appears to be a stimulant for appetite and feeding. It is also a strong stimulant of growth hormone secretion and has important direct cardiovascular effects. In addition, ghrelin has potent independent vasodilator properties.

GLUCOSE METER: A small, portable machine, used to check blood glucose levels.

GLUCONEOGENESIS: The formation of glucose from nutrients that are not themselves carbohydrates, as from amino acids, lactate, and fats.

GLUCOSE: A simple sugar that is the body's main source of energy, glucose is obtained through the breakdown of food in the digestive system.

GLYCEMIC INDEX (GI): A ranking system of carbohydrates according to their effect on blood glucose levels.

GLYCEMIC LOAD (GL): Glycemic load is the total amount of glucose delivered by the meal. To calculate the glycemic load, multiply the Glycemic Index of the food by the number of grams of available (total carbohydrate minus the fiber) carbohydrate and divide by 100.

GRAIN: Grain is composed of three layers. The **bran** is the fibrous outer layer that has most of the grain's minerals. The **endosperm** is the middle layer, comprising about 85 percent of a whole grain by weight. It contains mostly complex carbohydrates, along with small amounts of B vitamins. The **germ** is the smallest of the three components. It is a rich source of trace minerals, unsaturated fats, B vitamins, vitamin E, antioxidants, and phytonutrients. Whole grain has all three layers to contribute to the food's nutrition. Some processing removes the bran and other processing also removes the germ.

GROWTH HORMONE (GH): A hormone, made in the anterior pituitary gland, which stimulates tissue and skeletal growth.

HEIRLOOM: A plant that was developed and in cultivation sometime in the past and that is currently being maintained because of its desirable qualities.

HORMESIS: The stimulating or beneficial effect of small doses of a toxic substance or other biological stress, such as calorie restriction, that at higher doses has an inhibitory or adverse effect. Hormesis has been found in a wide variety of life forms—including human beings.

HORMONE: A chemical substance involved in the regulation and coordination of cellular and bodily functions.

HULLED AND HULL-LESS BARLEY: Hulled barley has been processed so minimally as to remove the outer chaff that it is still considered a whole grain. Hull-less barley is a different variety that grows without a hull; it needs no processing. Both increase the texture of any dish they are served in and provide fiber and a delightfully low GI.

HYPOGLYCEMIA: Low blood sugar, occurs when your blood glucose level drops too low to provide enough energy for your body's activities. It causes confusion, abnormal behavior, or both, such as the inability to complete routine tasks. Other symptoms may include visual disturbances, such as double vision and blurred vision, tremor, anxiety, sweating, hunger, heart palpitations, seizures, uncommon loss of consciousness. See your doctor if symptoms of hypoglycemia persist. Hypoglycemia can be an indication of potentially serious illness.

IGF-I—INSULIN-LIKE GROWTH FACTOR-I IGF-I: is important for carbohydrate and lipid metabolism and for the regulation of Growth Hormone secretion.

INFLAMMATION: The nonspecific immune response that occurs in reaction to any type of bodily injury. It is the same response whether the injuring agent is a pathogenic organism, foreign body, reduced blood flow, physical trauma, ionizing radiation, electrical energy, or extremes of temperature. The hallmarks of inflammation are pain, redness, swelling, heat, and often loss of function.

The reactions produced during inflammation and repair may be harmful, e.g., hypersensitivity reactions and the processes that lead to rheumatoid arthritis.

INSULIN: A hormone secreted by the pancreas that plays a major role in the regulation of glucose metabolism.

INSULIN-LIKE GROWTH FACTOR-I: *See* IGF-I.

KETOACIDOSIS: A severe condition characterized by high blood-glucose levels and ketones in the urine. It is caused by a lack of insulin or an elevation in stress hormones and occurs most often in those with Type 1 diabetes—when the liver lacks glucose but needs metabolic fuel, so it metabolizes fat and proteins.

KETONE BODIES: Any of three compounds that are produced as by-products when fatty acids are broken down for energy—they are used as a source of energy in various tissues including muscles, heart, renal cortex, kidney, and brain. In the brain, they are a vital energy source during fasting.

The three types of ketone bodies are acetoacetate, beta-hydroxybutyrate, and acetone. Only beta-hydroxybutyrate is produced in normal, healthy human beings at levels high enough to measure.

LAB TEST UNITS OF MEASURE—The following units of measure are commonly used for lab tests.

- IU—International Unit: the amount of a substance, such as insulin, that produces a specific effect as defined by an international body and accepted internationally
- mg/dl—milligrams (1/1000 of a gram) per deciliter (1/10 of a liter)
- mg/L—milligrams (1/1000 of a gram) per liter
- mIU/L—1/1000 of an International Unit per liter
- mIU/ml—1/1000 of an International Unit per milliliter (1/1000 of a liter)
- mmHg—millimeters of mercury in a sphygmomanometer, used to measure blood pressure
- mmol—millimole, a measurement of the concentration of chemicals in the body
- µg/dl—micrograms (one millionth of a gram) per deciliter (1/10 of a liter)
- µIU/ml—microIU per milliliter (one millionth of an International Unit per milliliter (1/1000 of a liter)
- ng/dl—nanogram (one billionth of a gram) per deciliter
- pg/ml—picograms (one trillionth of a gram) per milliliter (1/1000 of a liter)

LACTOBACILLUS ACIDOPHILUS: May be considered a probiotic or "friendly" bacterium. These types of healthy bacteria inhabit the intestines and vagina and protect against some unhealthy organisms.

LACTOSE: Sugar found in milk.

LYMPHATIC SYSTEM: A complex network of *organs*, nodes, ducts, tissues, capillaries, and vessels that produce and transport lymph fluid from tissues to the circulatory system.

The lymphatic system has three interrelated functions:

(1) removal of excess fluids from body tissues
(2) absorption of fatty acids and subsequent transport of fat to the circulatory system
(3) production of immune cells (such as lymphocytes)

MEDITATION: Mental practice that brings about calmness and physical relaxation by suspending the stream of thoughts that normally occupy the mind.

METABOLISM: All of the chemical changes that take place in living organisms; these changes include both production and breakdown of body constituents. More narrowly, they are the physical and chemical changes that take place in a given chemical substance within an organism. Metabolism includes the uptake and distribution within the body of chemical compounds, the changes (biotransformations) undergone by these substances, and the elimination of the compounds and their metabolites.

MITOCHONDRIA: Distinct bodies within cells that generate the power for the cells' chemical reactions.

MONOUNSATURATED FATTY ACIDS: Fatty acids with one double-bonded carbon in the molecule. Monounsaturated fats are found in many foods such as olive oil, peanuts, and avocados.

NEURON: Unique type of cell found in the brain and nervous system that is specialized to receive and transmit information.

NEUROTRANSMITTERS: Chemicals that facilitate communication between nerve cells, and are thought to play an important role in a person's feelings, emotions, actions, and behavior.

NITRIC OXIDE: In the body, nitric oxide is involved in oxygen transport to the tissues, the transmission of nerve impulses, and other physiological activities. The endothelium (inner lining) of blood vessels uses nitric oxide to signal the surrounding smooth muscle to relax, thus dilating the artery and increasing blood flow. Nitric oxide is also generated by macrophages and neutrophils as part of the human immune response. Nitric oxide is toxic to bacteria and other human pathogens.

NUTRIENT-DENSE: Descriptive of a food that has a high amount of nutrients per calorie.

NUTRIENTS: Compounds in foods that provide the nourishment that is essential for life. Nutrients include carbohydrates, proteins, fats, vitamins, and minerals.

OMEGA FATTY ACIDS: Omega fatty acids are known as essential fatty acids; they are essential to human health, but cannot be manufactured by the body and must be obtained from food.

Omega-3 fatty acids are found in nuts, seeds, fish oils of herring, mackerel, salmon, and sardines, as well as human breast milk. Omega-3 fatty acids include:

- α-linolenic acid (**ALA**),
- eicosapentaenoic acid (**EPA**)
- docosahexaenoic acid (**DHA**)

Omega-6 fatty acids are obtained in the diet from nuts, seeds, meat, eggs, and plants. Omega-6 fatty acids include:

- linoleic acid (**LA**)
- gamma-linolenic acid (**GLA**)
- arachidonic acid (**AA**)

ONCOGENE: A gene that normally directs cell growth—if altered, it can promote or allow the uncontrolled growth of cancer. Alterations can be inherited or caused by an environmental exposure to carcinogens.

ONCOGENIC: Giving rise to either benign or malignant tumors or causing tumor formation; said especially of tumor-inducing viruses.

ORTHOLOG: A gene with similar function to a gene in an evolutionarily related species.

ORTHOLOGOUS: Refers to a gene that has evolved from an ancestral gene.

OSTEOPOROSIS: Literally, porous bone. Abnormally reduced bone mass (density), which predisposes a person to fractures. As weight is lost, the bones tend to lose density, increasing the likelihood of osteoporosis. Food selection, exercise, and maintaining a healthy weight can counteract the bone-loss effect.

OXIDATION: The process of a chemical combination with oxygen. On the cellular level, oxidative reactions are the source of energy, but free radicals and other **oxidative residue** can damage cellular components, such as membranes, and interfere with cells' regulatory systems. (*See also* REACTIVE OXYGEN MOLECULES.)

PHYTOCHEMICAL: Plant substances known to have beneficial health effects.

PPAR-GAMMA—PEROXISOME: PROLIFERATOR-ACTIVATED RECEPTOR GAMMA: The body's master regulator of fat development.

PH: A measure of the acidity or alkalinity of a solution. Acidic solutions have a pH less than 7, while basic (alkaline) solutions have a pH greater than 7.

PLAQUE: Buildup of fatty deposits within the wall of a blood vessel.

PLASMA: Colorless watery fluid of blood and lymph containing no cells and in which red blood cells, white blood cells, and platelets are suspended.

POLYUNSATURATED FAT: A type of fat that is found in large amounts in foods from animals and plants, including safflower, sunflower, and corn oils.

PROBIOTIC: "Beneficial bacteria" that are cultured in laboratory conditions and are then used to restore the balance of the microflora (natural microbial resident population of the digestive system).

PROTEIN: The major structural component of all body tissue; necessary for muscular growth and cellular repair, proteins are also a functional component of enzymes, hormones, etc. They are used for energy only when carbohydrates and fats are not available.

PROTEIN DIGESTIBILITY CORRECTED AMINO ACID SCORE (PDCAAS): A method of evaluating protein quality—the PDCAAS rating was adopted by the U.S. Food and Drug Administration (FDA) and the Food and Agricultural Organization of the United Nations/World Health Organization (FAO/WHO) in 1993. Because the PDCAAS is based on the amino acid **requirements** of humans, 100 percent or 1.00 is the highest possible score. A score of 1.00 indicates that the protein contains essential amino acids in excess of the human requirements.

While the originating agencies have not come forward with additional values to replace the 1.00 score, independent evaluations have corroborated the need for them. Research* by and outside of these agencies shows that an egg has a score of 1.18 and cow's milk, 1.21. Further research† has shown that whey has a score of 1.14 on a scale on which egg came in at 1.00. We have calculated whey's PDCAAS for the FAO/WHO scale for comparison purposes. Although this is not the ideal methodology, the values do provide the opportunity for ranking the proteins' *availability*.

REACTIVE OXYGEN MOLECULES, or REACTIVE OXYGEN SPECIES (ROS): Unstable, highly reactive molecules that react with anything they contact such as cells or the DNA. For a long time it was thought that ROS were only damaging, but it is now known that ROS play beneficial roles in the body such as vasodilation.

Reactive oxygen molecules are produced continuously in all air-breathing animals, including humans. These molecules are a by-

---

*FAO/WHO Expert consultation (1990). Protein Quality Evaluation. Food and Agriculture Organization of the United Nations, Food and Nutrition Paper 51, Rome; European Dairy Association (1997) Nutritional Quality of Proteins, Brussels, Belgium; E. Renner (1983). Milk and Dairy Products in Human Nutrition. W-Gmbh Volkswirtschlaftlicher, München, pp. 90–130.

†Reported by Whey Research, Carlsbad, CA. http://www.wheyresearch.com/what iswhey.php. Accessed March 18, 2007.

product of normal metabolism. Because the normal metabolic path depends on the consumption and chemical use of oxygen, the production of ROS is unavoidable.

RED BLOOD CELL: Blood cell that contains and carries oxygen through the bloodstream to organs and tissues and carbon dioxide away from them for disposal.

RESVERATROL: A substance that is produced in plants in response to an invading fungus, stress, injury, infection, or ultraviolet irradiation. Resveratrol is contained in grapes, raspberries, peanuts, and numerous other plants. Resveratrol has been shown to be a potent stimulator of the longevity gene, SIRT-1.

SATURATED FAT: A fat that is solid at room temperature and is found in foods from animal meats and skin, dairy products, and some vegetables. Studies show that too much saturated fat in a person's diet increases heart disease risk.

SAVORING MEDITATION: A contemplative enjoyment of small portions of food.

SEROTONIN: A hormone found in the brain, platelets, digestive tract, and pineal gland. It acts both as a neurotransmitter (a substance that nerves use to send messages) and a vasoconstrictor (a substance that causes blood vessels to narrow). A lack of serotonin in the brain is thought to be a cause of depression.

SIR—SILENT INFORMATION REGULATOR: A gene that regulates the deactivation or "silencing" of other cell signaling.

SIRTUINS: Sirtuins is a conserved family of proteins found in all domains of life. The first known sirtuin, Sir2 (silent information regulator 2) of yeast, from which the family derives its name, regulates ribosomal DNA recombination, gene silencing, DNA repair, chromosomal stability, and longevity. Sir2 homologues also modulate life span in worms and flies, and may underlie the beneficial effects of calorie restriction.

A family of seven (so far identified) genes, found in humans. In mammals, the homologous genes are called SIRT1 through SIRT7, where the T stands for 2, reducing the confusion of two numerals beside each other. Biological functions ranging from DNA repair to metabolism regulation are associated with six of the seven sirtuins found in mammals. SIRT1, SIRT3, and SIRT4 have been shown to play key roles in regulating metabolism in response to dietary changes.

SIRT1: The most researched of the genes in the sirtuin family. It is thought to play an important role in the beneficial biological changes brought about by calorie restriction.

SOFTNESS MEDITATION: Meditation that focuses on progressive relaxation of the body for the purpose of inducing sleep.

SUCROSE: Table sugar, also called "saccharose."

TEASE MEAL: A single, small course, eaten before the main meal, for the purpose of activating insulin production.

TESTOSTERONE: The male hormone, made primarily in the testes. It stimulates blood flow, growth in certain tissues, and the secondary sexual characteristics. In men with prostate cancer, it can also encourage growth of the tumor. Small amounts of testosterone are also produced in women by the ovaries and the adrenal glands.

TOR—"TARGET OF RAPAMYCIN": An enzyme complex, named

after the drug rapamycin that deactivates it, its activity regulates cell size and growth. The acronym also appears as (m)TOR for (mammalian)TOR.

TRIGLYCERIDES: The chemical form in which most fat exists in food as well as in the body. They are also present in blood plasma and, in association with cholesterol, constitute the lipids circulating in the blood.

Triglycerides in plasma are derived from fats eaten in foods or made in the body from other energy sources, like carbohydrates. Calories ingested in a meal and not used immediately by tissues are converted to triglycerides and transported to fat cells to be stored. Hormones regulate the release of triglycerides from fat tissue so they meet the body's needs for energy between meals.

TRYPTOPHAN: An amino acid that occurs in proteins, is essential for growth and normal metabolism, and is a precursor of niacin, which helps the body produce serotonin, a chemical that acts as a calming agent in the brain and plays a role in sleep.

VAP—VERTICAL AUTO PROFILE TEST: A comprehensive lipoprotein risk assessment for total cholesterol/lipid management.

WHITE BLOOD CELLS: A variety of cells that, as part of the immune system, fight infection in the body.

APPENDIX F

BIBLIOGRAPHY

Abdallah L, Chabert M, Louis-Sylvestre J. **Cephalic phase responses to sweet taste.** *American Journal of Clinical Nutrition.* **1997** Mar;65(3):737–43. PMID: 9062523

Abrahamson PE, Gammon MD, Lund MJ, Flagg EW, Porter PL, et al. **General and abdominal obesity and survival among young women with breast cancer.** *Cancer Epidemiology, Biomarkers and Prevention.* **2006** Oct;15(10):1871–7. PMID: 17035393

Ahren B, Holst JJ. **The cephalic insulin response to meal ingestion in humans is dependent on both cholinergic and noncholinergic mechanisms and is important for postprandial glycemia.** *Diabetes.* 2001 May;50(5):1030–8. PMID: 11334405

Alexander CN, Langer EJ, Newman RI, Chandler HM, Davies JL. **Transcendental meditation, mindfulness, and longevity: an experimental study with the elderly.** *J Pers Soc Psychol.* 1989 Dec;57(6):950–64. PMID: 2693686

Alssema M, Dekker JM, Nijpels G, Stehouwer CD, Bouter LM, Heine RJ; Hoorn Study. **Proinsulin concentration is an independent predictor of all-cause and cardiovascular mortality: an 11-year follow-up of the Hoorn Study.** *Diabetes Care.* 2005 Apr;28(4):860–5. PMID: 15793186 http://care.diabetesjournals.org/cgi/content/full/28/4/860, accessed June 28, 2007

American Heart Association, **Cholesterol Levels: AHA Recommendation,** http://www.americanheart.org/presenter.jhtml?identifier=4500, accessed Sept. 11, 2007

Andres-Lacueva C, Shukitt-Hale B, Galli RL, Jauregui O, Lamuela-Raventos RM, Joseph JA. **Anthocyanins in aged blueberry-fed rats are found centrally and may enhance memory.** *Nutritional Neuroscience.* **2005** Apr;8(2):111–20. PMID: 16053243

Baur JA, Pearson KJ, Price NL, Jamieson HA, Sinclair DA, et al. **Resveratrol improves health and survival of mice on a high-calorie diet.** *Nature.* **2006** Nov 16; 444 (7117):337–42. PMID: 17086191

Behall KM, Scholfield DJ, Hallfrisch J. **Diets containing barley significantly reduce lipids in mildly hypercholesterolemic men and women.** *American Journal of Clinical Nutrition.* **2004** Nov;80(5):1185–93

Benson H. *Beyond the Relaxation Response.* New York: Times Books, **1984**

Bernstein, RK. *Dr. Bernstein's Diabetes Solution: A Complete Guide to Achieving Normal Blood Sugars.* Boston: Little, Brown & Co., **1997**, especially p. 253

Boyd DB. **Insulin and cancer.** *Integrative Cancer Therapy.* **2003** Dec;2(4):315–29. PMID: 14713323

Bruce DG, Storlien LH, Furler SM, Chisholm DJ. **Cephalic phase metabolic responses in normal weight adults.** *Metabolism.* **1987** Aug;36(8):721–5. PMID: 3298939

Bui T, Thompson CB. **Cancer's sweet tooth.** *Cancer Cell.* **2006** Jun;9(6):419–20. PMID: 16766260

Carter J, et al. Body composition of Montreal Olympics Athletes In: *Physical structure of Olympic athletes.* Part I. Ed: JEL Carter. Basel: Karger, **1982**, 107–116

Centers for Disease Control and Prevention. **BMI CHARTS.** http://www .cdc.gov/nccdphp/dnpa/bmi/adult_BMI/about_adult_BMI.htm# Definition, accessed 3-2-**2007**

Chen J, Zhou Y, Mueller-Steiner S, Chen LF, Kwon H, Yi S, et al. **SIRT1 protects against microglia-dependent beta amyloid toxicity through inhibiting NF-kappa B signaling.** *J Biol Chem.* **2005** Sep 23. PMID: 16183991

Chlebowski RT, Aiello E, McTiernan A. **Weight loss in breast cancer patient management.** *Journal of Clinical Oncology.* **2002** Feb 15;20(4):1128–43. PMID: 11844838

Civitarese AE, Carling C, Heilbronn HK, Hulver MH, Ukropcova B, Deutsch WA, Smith SR, Ravussin, E; CALERIE Pennington Team. **Calorie** restriction increases muscle mitochondrial biogenesis in healthy humans. *PLOS Med.* 2007 Mar;4(3):e76, PMID: 17341128

Cohen HY, Miller C, Bitterman KJ, Wall NR, Sinclair DA, et al. Calorie restriction promotes mammalian cell survival by inducing the SIRT1 deacetylase. *Science.* 2004 Jul 16;305(5682):390–2. Epub 2004 Jun 17. PMID: 15205477

Cortes B, Núñez I, Cofan M, Gilabert R, Perez-Heras A, et al. Acute effects of high-fat meals enriched with walnuts or olive oil on postprandial endothelial function. *Journal of the American College of Cardiology.* 2006 Oct 17;48(8):1666–71. PMID: 17045905

Delarue J, Labarthe F, Cohen R. Fish-oil supplementation reduces stimulation of plasma glucose fluxes during exercise in untrained males. *British Journal of Nutrition.* 2003 Oct;90(4):777–86. PMID: 13129446

Dew MA, Hoch CC, Buysse DJ, Monk TH, Begley AE, et al. Healthy older adults' sleep predicts all-cause mortality at 4 to 19 years of follow-up. *Psychosomatic Medicine.* 2003 Jan–Feb;65(1):63–73. PMID: 12554816

Dhahbi JM, Mote PL, Wingo J, Tillman JB, Walford RL, Spindler SR. Calories and aging alter gene expression for gluconeogenic, glycolytic, and nitrogen-metabolizing enzymes. *American Journal of Physiology* 1999 Aug;277 (2 Pt 1):E352–60 PMID: 10444432

DIET DETECTIVE® The health and fitness network, © 2007–2008. Integrated Wellness Solutions Corp. http://dietdetective.com/, accessed 3-1-2007

Dobbins RL, Chester MW, Daniels MB, McGarry JD, Stein DT. Circulating fatty acids are essential for efficient glucose-stimulated insulin secretion after prolonged fasting in humans. *Diabetes.* 1998 Oct;47(10): 1613–8. PMID: 9753300

Duelli R, Staudt R, Duembgen L, Kuschinsky W. Increase in glucose transporter densities of Glut3 and decrease of glucose utilization in rat brain after one week of hypoglycemia. *Brain Research.* 1999 Jun 12;831(1–2):254–62. PMID: 10412004

Elias PK, Elias MF, D'Agostino RB, Sullivan LM, Wolf PA. Serum cholesterol and cognitive performance in the Framingham Heart Study. *Psychosomatic Medicine.* 2005 Jan–Feb;67(1):24–30. PMID: 15673620

Engelberg H. Low serum cholesterol and suicide. *Lancet.* 1992 Mar 21;339(8795):727. PMID: 1347593

Epel ES, Blackburn EH, Lin J, Dhabhar FS, Adler NE, et al. Accelerated telomere shortening in response to life stress. *Proceedings of the National Academy of Sciences.* 2004 Dec 14;101(50):17323–4. PMID: 15574496

Feldeisen SE, Tucker KL. **Nutritional strategies in the prevention and treatment of metabolic syndrome.** *Applied Physiology, Nutrition and Metabolism.* 2007 Feb;32(1):46–60. PMID: 17332784

Fontana L, Meyer TE, Klein S, Holloszy JO. **Long-term calorie restriction is highly effective in reducing the risk for atherosclerosis in humans.** *Proceedings of the National Academy of Sciences of the USA.* 2004 101 (17): 6659–63. PMID: 15096581

Fontana L, Klein S, Holloszy JO. **Long-term low-protein, low-calorie diet and endurance exercise modulate metabolic factors associated with cancer risk.** *American Journal of Clinical Nutrition.* 2006 Dec;84(6):1456–62. PMID: 17158430

Fontana L, Klein S. **Aging, adiposity, and calorie restriction.** *Journal of the American Medical Association* 2007. Mar 7;297(9):986–94. Review. PMID: 17341713

Frid AH, Nilsson M, Holst JJ, Bjorck IM. **Effect of whey on blood glucose and insulin responses to composite breakfast and lunch meals in type 2 diabetic subjects.** *American Journal of Clinical Nutrition.* 2005 Jul;82(1):69–75. PMID:16002802

Galeone C, Pelucchi C, Levi F, Negri E, Franceschi S, et al. **Onion and garlic use and human cancer.** *American Journal of Clinical Nutrition.* 2006 Nov;84(5):1027–32. PMID: 17093154

Gannon MC, Ercan N, Westphal SA, Nuttall FQ. **Effect of added fat on plasma glucose and insulin response to ingested potato in individuals with NIDDM.** *Diabetes Care.* 1993 Jun;16(6):874–80. PMID: 8325201

Ganong, William F. **Hypothalmic control of growth hormone secretion, and endocrine functions of the pancreas and regulation of carbohydrate metabolism: protein and fat derivatives.** *Review of Medical Physiology.* New York: Lange Medical Books/McGraw-Hill, 21st edition, 2003

Ganong, William F. *Review of Medical Physiology.* New York: Lange Medical Books/McGraw-Hill, 22nd edition, 2005

Goldberg T, Cai W, Peppa M, Dardaine V, Baliga BS, Uribarri J. **Advanced glycoxidation end products in commonly consumed foods.** *Journal of the American Dietetic Association.* 2005 Apr;105(4):647. PMID: 15281050

Golier JA, Marzuk PM, Leon AC, Weiner C, Tardiff K. **Low serum** cholesterol level and attempted suicide. *American Journal of Psychiatry.* **1995**; 152: 419–23. PMID: 7864269

Halkjaer J, Tjonneland A, Thomsen BL, Overvad K, Sorensen TI. Intake of macronutrients as predictors of 5-y changes in waist circumference. *American Journal of Clinical Nutrition.* **2006** Oct;84(4):789–97. PMID: 17023705

Hammes HP, Du X, Edelstein D, Taguchi T, Matsumura T, et al. Benfotiamine blocks three major pathways of hyperglycemic damage and prevents experimental diabetic retinopathy. *Nature Medicine* **2003** Mar;9(3):294–9. PMID: 12592403

Hsieh EA, Chai CM, Hellerstein MK. Effects of caloric restriction on cell proliferation in several tissues in mice: role of intermittent feeding. *American Journal of Physiology, Endocrinology and Metabolism.* **2005** May;288(5):E965–72. PMID: 15613681

Hursting SD, Lavigne JA, Berrigan D, Perkins SN, Barrett JC. Calorie restriction, aging, and cancer prevention: mechanisms of action and applicability to humans. *Annual Review of Medicine.* **2003**;54:131–52. Review. PMID: 12525670

Kashiwaya Y, Takeshima T, Mori N, Nakashima K, Clarke K, Veech RL. D-beta-hydroxybutyrate protects neurons in models of Alzheimer's and Parkinson's disease. *Proceedings of the National Academy of Sciences.* **2000** May 9;97(10):5440–4. PMID: 10805800

Koschinsky T, He CJ, Mitsuhashi T, Bucala R, Liu C, Buenting C, Heitmann K. Orally absorbed reactive glycation products (glycotoxins): an environmental risk factor in diabetic nephropathy. *Proceedings of the National Academy of Sciences.* **1997** Jun 10;94(12):6474–9. PMID: 9177242

Kuk JL, Katzmarzyk PT, Nichaman MZ, Church TS, Blair SN, Ross R. Visceral fat is an independent predictor of all-cause mortality in men. *Obesity* (Silver Spring). **2006** Feb;14(2):336–41. PMID: 16571861

Lamers KJ, Gabreëls FJ, Renier WO, Wevers RA, Doesburg WH. Fasting studies in cerebrospinal fluid and blood in children with epilepsy of unknown origin. *Epilepsy Research.* **1995** May;21(1):59–63. PMID: 7641677

Larsson SC, Bergkvist L, Wolk A. Consumption of sugar and sugar-sweetened foods and the risk of pancreatic cancer in a prospective study. *American Journal of Clinical Nutrition* **2006** Nov;84(5):1171–6

Lau FC, Shukitt-Hale B, Joseph JA. The beneficial effects of fruit polyphenols on brain aging. *Neurobiology of Aging.* **2005** Dec;26 Suppl 1:128–32: PMID: 16194581

Lazar SW, Kerr CE, Wasserman RH, Gray JR, Greve DN, et al. **Meditation experience is associated with increased cortical thickness.** *Neuroreport.* **2005** Nov 28;16(17):1893–7. PMID: 16272874

Lee IM, Manson JE, Hennekens CH, Paffenbarger RS. **Body weight and mortality. A 27-year follow-up of middle-aged men.** *Journal of the American Medical Association.* **1993** Dec 15; 270(23): 2823–8. PMID: 8133621

Lehninger AL, Nelson DL, Cox MM. *Principles of Biochemistry.* New York: Worth Publishers, 4th ed. **2004,** especially first-phase insulin

Levi B, Werman MJ. **Long-term fructose consumption accelerates glycation and several age-related variables in male rats.** *Journal of Nutrition.* **1998** Sep;128(9):1442–9. PMID: 9732303

Lopez-Lluch G, Hunt N, Jones B, Zhu M, Jamieson H, Hilmer S, et al. **Calorie restriction induces mitochondrial biogenesis and bioenergetic efficiency.** *Proceedings of the National Academy of Sciences.* **2006** Feb 7;103(6): 1768–73. Epub **2006** Jan 30. PMID: 16446459

Lutz A, Greischar LL, Rawlings NB, Richard M, Davidson RJ. **Long-term meditators self-induce high-amplitude gamma synchrony during mental practice.** *Proceedings of the National Academy of Sciences.* **2004** Nov 16;101(46):16369–73. PMID: 15534199

Maalouf M, Sullivan PG, Davis L, Kim DY, Rho JM. **Ketones inhibit mitochondrial production of reactive oxygen species production following glutamate excitotoxicity by increasing NADH oxidation.** *Neuroscience.* **2007** Mar 2;145(1):256–64. PMID: 17240074

Macho A, Lucena C, Sancho R, Daddario N, Minassi A, Muñoz E, Appendino G. **Non-pungent capsaicinoids from sweet pepper synthesis and evaluation of the chemopreventive and anticancer potential.** *European Journal of Nutrition* **2003** Jan;42(1):2–9. PMID: 12594536

Mackowiak PA, Wasserman SS, Levine MM. **A critical appraisal of 98.6 degrees F, the upper limit of the normal body temperature, and other legacies of Carl Reinhold August Wunderlich.** *JAMA: the Journal of the American Medical Association.* **1992** Sep 23–30;268(12):1578–80. PMID: 1302471

Manson JE. **Body weight and longevity. A reassessment.** *Journal of the American Medical Association.* **1987** Jan 16;257(3):353–8. PMID: 3795418

Manson JE, Willett WC, Stampfer MJ, Colditz GA, Hunter DJ, Manson E, et al. **Body weight and mortality among women.** *New England Journal of Medicine.* **1995** Sep 14;333(11):677–85. PMID: 7637744

Masoro, EJ. **Calorie restriction: a key to understanding and modulating aging,** *(Research Profiles in Aging).* Amsterdam: Elsevier, **2002.**

Mattison JA, Lane MA, Roth GS, Ingram DK. **Calorie restriction in rhesus monkeys.** *Experimental Gerontology.* **2003** Jan–Feb;38(1–2):35–46. PMID: 12543259

Mattson MP. **Neuroprotective signaling and the aging brain: take away my food and let me run.** *Brain Research.* **2000** Dec 15;886(1–2):47–53. PMID: 11119686

Mattson MP, Duan W, Guo Z. **Meal size and frequency affect neuronal plasticity and vulnerability to disease: cellular and molecular mechanisms.** *Journal of Neurochemistry.* **2003** Feb;84(3):417–31. PMID: 12558961

McGlothin P. **Savoring meditation.** *CR IV* (Fourth Conference of the Calorie Restriction Society. April 7 and 8. **2006** April 5 to 9, Tucson, AZ)

McPherson JD, Shilton BH, Walton DJ. **Role of fructose in glycation and cross-linking of proteins.** *Biochemistry.* **1988** Mar 22;27(6):1901–7. PMID: 3132203

Meyer TE, Kovacs SJ, Ehsani AA, Klein S, Holloszy JO, Fontana L. **Long-term caloric restriction ameliorates the decline in diastolic function in humans.** *Journal of American College of Cardiology.* **2006** Jan 17;47(2):398–402. PMID: 16412867

Michels KB, Ekbom A. **Caloric restriction and incidence of breast cancer.** *Journal of the American Medical Association.* **2004** Mar 10;291(10):1226–30. (Swedish breast cancer study) PMID: 15010444

Monteleone P, Maj M, Fusco M, Orazzo C, Kemali D. **Physical exercise at night blunts the nocturnal increase of plasma melatonin levels in healthy humans.** *Life Sciences.* **1990**;47(22):1989–95. PMID: 2273939

National Heart, Lung and Blood Institute, *The Fourth Report on the Diagnosis, Evaluation, and Treatment of High Blood Pressure in Children and Adolescents,* NIH Publication 05–5267, originally printed Sept **1996** (96–3790), revised May **2005**

NIH, CDC, and DHHS **Body weight, health and longevity: conclusions and recommendations of the workshop.** *Nutrition Reviews,* **1985** Feb; 43(2), 61–3. PMID: 3991081

Nagaya N, Kangawa K. **Therapeutic potential of ghrelin in the treatment of heart failure.** *Drugs.* **2006**;66 (4):439–48. PMID: 16597162

Nielsen NR, Thygesen LC, Johansen D, Jensen G, Grønbaek M. The influence of duration of follow-up on the association between alcohol and cause-specific mortality in a prospective cohort study. *Annals of Epidemiology.* 2005 Jan;15(1):44–55. PMID: 15571993

Oliver SE, Barrass B, Gunnell DJ., Donovan JL, Peters TJ, et al. Serum insulin-like growth factor-I is positively associated with serum prostate-specific antigen in middle-aged men without evidence of prostate cancer. *Cancer Epidemiology, Biomarkers & Prevention.* 2004 Jan;13(1):163–5. PMID: 14744750

Pedersen BK, Rohde T, Ostrowski K. Recovery of the immune system after exercise. *Acta Physiologica Scandinavica.* 1998 Mar;162(3):325–32. Review. PMID: 9578378

Picard F, Guarente L. Molecular links between aging and adipose tissue. *International Journal of Obesity* (London). 2005 Mar;29 Suppl 1:S36–9. PMID: 15711582

Picard F, Kurtev M, Chung N, Topark-Ngarm A, Guarente L, et al. SIRT1 promotes fat mobilization in white adipocytes by repressing PPAR-gamma. *Nature.* 2004 Jun 17;429(6993):771–6. Epub 2004 Jun 2 PMID: 15175761

Reger MA, Henderson ST, Hale C, Cholerton B, Baker LD, et al. Effects of b-hydroxybutyrate on cognition in memory-impaired adults. *Neurobiology of Aging.* 2004 Mar;25(3):311–4. PMID: 15123336

Richardson A, Portwood M. The Durham (England) trial on EPA's and DHA's effect on cognitive performance in children. Department of Physiology at Mansfield College, University of Oxford, and Special-Education Psychology at Durham Local Education Authority. 2007 In press.

Rodgers JT, Lerin C, Haas W, Gygi SP, Spiegelman BM, Puigserver P. Nutrient control of glucose homeostasis through a complex of PGC-1alpha and SIRT1. *Nature.* 2005 Mar 3;434(7029):113–8. PMID: 15744310

Rodriguez BL, Lau N, Burchfiel CM, Abbott RD, Sharp DS, et al. Glucose intolerance and 23-year risk of coronary heart disease and total mortality: the Honolulu Heart Program. *Diabetes Care.* 1999 Aug;22(8):1262–5. PMID: 10480768

Roth GS, Lesnikov V, Lesnikov M, Ingram DK, Lane, MA. Dietary caloric restriction prevents the age-related decline in plasma melatonin levels of rhesus monkeys. *Journal of Clinical Endocrinology and Metabolism.* 2001 Jul;86(7):3292–5. PMID: 11443203

Rubio-Viqueira B, Hidalgo M. **Targeting mTOR for cancer treatment.** *Advances Experimental Medicine and Biology.* **2006**;587:309–27. PMID: 17163174

Sato K, Kashiwaya Y, Keon CA, Tsuchiya N, Veech RL, et al. **Insulin, ketone bodies, and mitochondrial energy transduction.** *FASEB Journal.* **1995** May;9(8):651–8. (Federation of American Societies for Experimental Biology) PMID: 7768357

Muchan S, Sinclair D. **Sirtuins in mammals: insights into their biological function.** *Biochemical Journal.* **2007** May 15;404(1):1–13. Review. PMID: 17447894

Sharma V, McNeill JH. **The emerging roles of leptin and ghrelin in cardiovascular physiology and pathophysiology.** *Current Vascular Pharmacology.* **2005** Apr;3(2):169–80. PMID: 15853636

Shirayama Y, Chen AC, Nakagawa S, Russell DS, Duman RS. **Brain-derived neurotrophic factor produces antidepressant effects in behavioral models of depression.** *Journal of Neuroscience.* **2002** Apr 15;22(8):3251–61. PMID: 11943826

Sinclair DA. **Toward a unified theory of caloric restriction and longevity regulation.** *Mechanisms of Ageing and Development.* **2005** Sep;126(9): 987–1002. PMID: 15893363

Singh RB, Niaz MA, Beegom R, Wander GS, Thakur AS, Rissam HS. **Body fat percent by bioelectrical impedance analysis and risk of coronary artery disease among urban men with low rates of obesity: the Indian paradox.** *Journal of the American College of Nutrition.* **1999** Jun;18(3):268–73. PMID: 10376784

Snow CM, Shaw JM, Winters KM, Witzke KA. **Long-term exercise using weighted vests prevents hip bone loss in postmenopausal women.** *Journals of Gerontology Series A: Biological Sciences and Medical Sciences.* **2000** Sep;55(9):M489–91. PMID: 10995045

Solomon CG, Manson JE. **Obesity and mortality: a review of the epidemiologic data.** *American Journal of Clinical Nutrition.* **1997** Oct, 66(4 Suppl), 1044S–1050S. PMID: 9322585

Sonntag WE, Xu X, Ingram RL, D'Costa A. **Moderate caloric restriction alters the subcellular distribution of somatostatin mRNA and increases growth hormone pulse amplitude in aged animals.** *Neuroendocrinology.* **1995** May;61(5):601–8. PMID: 7617139

Spindler SR, Dhahbi JM. **Conserved and tissue-specific genic and physiologic responses to caloric restriction and altered IGF-I signaling in** mitotic and postmitotic tissues. *Annual Review of Nutrition*. 2007 Apr 11 [Epub ahead of print]. PMID: 17428180

Stirban A, Negrean M, Koschinsky T, Vlassara H, Tschoepe D, et al. Benfotiamine prevents macro- and microvascular endothelial dysfunction and oxidative stress following a meal rich in advanced glycation end products in individuals with type 2 diabetes. *Diabetes Care*. 2006 Sep;29(9):2064–71 PMID: 16936154

Storlien LH, Bruce DG. Mind over metabolism: the cephalic phase in relation to non-insulin-dependent diabetes and obesity. *Biological Psychology*. 1989 Feb;28(1):3–23 Review. PMID: 2675992

Terman A, Brunk UT. Oxidative stress, accumulation of biological "garbage," and aging. Antioxid Redox Signal. 2006 Jan–Feb;8(1–2):197–204. PMID: 16487053

Thiebaut AC, Kipnis V, Chang SC, Subar AF, Thompson FE, et al. Dietary fat and postmenopausal invasive breast cancer in the National Institutes of Health-AARP Diet and Health Study cohort. *Journal of the National Cancer Institute*. 2007 Mar 21;99(6):451–62. PMID: 17374835

U.S. Department of Health & Human Services. *Dietary Guidelines for Americans*, 2005, Figure 2, page 17, http://www.health.gov/dietaryguidelines/dga2005/document/pdf/DGA2005.pdf

University of Pennsylvania Health System, Encyclopedia: Internal Medicine, Weight Management. Reviewed By: Jonathan Harding, MD, CPE, Department of Medicine, University of Massachusetts Medical School, Worcester, MA. Review date: 11/15/2005 http://pennhealth.com/ency/article/001943.htm, accessed July. 8, 2007

Wikipedia, The Free Encyclopedia, **Ketone**, http://en.wikipedia.org/wiki/Ketone, accessed Jan. 29, 2007

Wilson MA, Shukitt-Hale B, Kalt W, Ingram DK, Joseph JA, Wolkow CA. Blueberry polyphenols increase life span and thermotolerance in Caenorhabditis elegans. *Aging Cell*. 2006 Feb;5(1):59–68. PMID: 16441844

World Health Organization Diabetes Programme. Prevalence of diabetes worldwide. 2007, http://www.who.int/diabetes/facts/world_figures/en/, accessed Jan. 6, 2007

Wu MS, Yu CC, Wu CH, Haung JY, Leu ML, Huang CC. Pre-dialysis glycemic control is an independent predictor of mortality in type II diabetic patients on continuous ambulatory peritoneal dialysis. *Peritoneal Dialysis International*. 1999;19 Suppl 2:S179–83. PMID: 10406515

Wurtman JJ. *Managing Your Mind and Mood Through Food.* New York: Harper & Row, Publishers, 1986.

Yaghmaie F, Saeed O, Garan SA, Voelker MA, Gouw AM, et al. Age-dependent loss of insulin-like growth factor-1 receptor immunoreactive cells in the supraoptic hypothalamus is reduced in calorically restricted mice. *International Journal of Developmetal Neuroscience.* 2006 Nov;24(7):431–6. Epub 2006 Oct 10. PMID: 17034982

Yang H, Yang T, Baur JA, Perez E, Matsui T, de Cabo R, Sinclair DA, et al. Nutrient-sensitive mitochondrial NAD+ levels dictate cell survival. *Cell.* 2007 Sep 21; 130(6):1095–107. PMID: 17889652

Yeung F, Hoberg JE, Ramsey CS, Keller MD, Jones DR, et al. Modulation of NF-κB-dependent transcription and cell survival by the SIRT1 deacetylase. *EMBO Journal.* 2004 Jun 16;23(12):2369–80 (European Molecular Biology Organization). PMID: 15152190

Youngman LD. Protein restriction (PR) and caloric restriction (CR) compared: effects on DNA damage, carcinogenesis, and oxidative damage. *Mutation Research.* 1993 Dec;295(4–6):165–79. PMID: 7507555

INDEX